GRIEFS SLIPPERY SLOPE

Mallory Mills

© Copyright Mallory Mills- All rights reserved.

It is not legal to reproduce, duplicate, or transmit any part of this document in either electronic means or printed format. Recording of this publication is strictly prohibited.

Table of Contents

DEFINE NORMAL 5
THE DREADED FLU 14
THE MAKING OF A MAN 41
WE ARE NOT DEALING WITH THE FLU! 48
SILENCE & SOLITUDE 69
THE FAMILY ROCKED 74
A MOMENT TO REMEMBER 77
WILL THAT BE A LA CARTE? 82
WHO MAKES PLANS? 94
DENIAL 97
RIPPLE EFFECT 102
THE CAVE DWELLER 106
TIDES OF CHANGE 109
RESISTING CHANGE WILL BREAK YOU! 111
ACCEPTING CHANGE 116
SOCIAL HAUNTING 127
HAPPY NEW YEAR 130
THE SUN THROUGH THE CLOUDS 132
A COMPANION DOES NOT MEAN I'M LOOKING FOR SEX! 139
JUST COFFEE 142
OUR DAILY PEP TALKS. 144
CROSSING THAT BRIDGE 147
BUILDING A NEW WALL 150

FINDING YOUR SQUAD 153
COMPARING APPLES TO ORANGES 157
MY HOPE IS TO LOVE YOU AGAIN! 161

DEFINE NORMAL

After Evan's passing, I do not know how many times a day I would ask myself, "when will my life finally be back to normal or even halfway normal, maybe even at a point where I no longer hated the world and all the fucking normal people in it!" I would look at families and instantly be jealous and angry at what they had! I wanted to say to them, "Look at you and your beautiful family! You are all just fucking perfect!. All of you are on vacation, smiling, laughing, and enjoying the beach together. Yeah, well, you know what, I had that at one time also. Enjoy it now because these happy, joyous moments do not last forever!"

There was no reason for me to be so angry and hateful with these people other than I no longer had a husband, and my children no longer had their father. I was angry at family, friends, and complete strangers. They were going to feel my pain. Every part of me disliked them! Those happy, smiling faces were killing me deep down inside. Every smile on their face reinforced the complete happiness they were feeling at that moment. I felt that my life had flatlined for eternity!

Each and every day would be a struggle and a reminder for me and the kids that Evan wasn't going to be walking through that front door ever again! In my mind, I felt the better I played the part of normal, the better off my kids would be emotionally. Even if that meant, in my world, I would continue to deny that Evan was gone. Suddenly, I was alone. I was the sole caregiver to our kids, and this was now all on my shoulders. Every decision, it was now me!

I did not want to see your happiness; I did not want to feel your emotions. It was inevitable I would someday be the one in the crowd somewhere watching you celebrate so many triumphs and milestones together as a family, graduations, weddings, and eventually enjoying your beautiful grandchildren. You will watch your senior graduate, their cap flying high in the air, and you will be filled with pride in his accomplishments.

You will feel happy, tearful emotions as you walk your daughter down the aisle. You will be the hero in your daughters' eyes as you dance your first father-daughter dance at her wedding.

Every one of you will go home, sit down at the table, and enjoy dinner as a family. Every one of you will sit in the living room watching a movie and laughing together. Some of you will hop in your car and go watch your kids at their sporting event. Not me. Not my family!

I could not bear to hear or respond to people when they asked me how I was doing. Honestly, right now, they were not going to get a truthful answer out of me. It was always, "I'm doing fine." As the days became sunny and warm and people would comment, "Isn't it a beautiful day?" Yes, it was a beautiful day in your world. I no longer felt grateful to be blessed with another beautiful day on earth. I would have people say, "Mallory, everything will get better with time." It was always amazing to hear this come from someone that never lost their spouse. These people had no clue. They never walked a day in my shoes but somehow knew with time, everything would be better. I would look at them and think, "Sure, you know, giving out all this helpful advice as your husband stands right next to you!"

The once strong, independent, and mentally thriving young woman was no longer present. Instead, a woman crippled by anxiety and fear of what was to come next and not sure how she was going to deal with it. That mom, which was always happy to participate in school functions and volunteer to help out when needed, now cringed at the thought of being around other people. That mom that welcomed her children's friends over now dreaded the idle chit-chat with parents at drop-off and pickup.

The invites to parties and events were so difficult, but not attending them would give my children the impression that something was wrong. I would get dressed, drag Bryan along, smile, and make small talk. I would do everything that would make it appear that I was socially engaged. The odd part about attending some of these events is how awkward people were towards Bryan and me. I know they wanted to say something, but sometimes they would just look at us from across the room with so much sadness in their eyes I almost got upset for them!

    I just do not think people realized how uncomfortable it was for me when they walked up to me, gave me a hug, and would say, "I'm so sorry to hear about Evan. How are you and the kids doing?" A smile is all I would offer back to them; it was not the time or the place for me. Honestly, just a hug would have sufficed, I would have known exactly what it was for!

    After a question like that, it was always difficult for me to get my mind out of that memory recycle mode. I would be the quiet zombie in the corner thinking about Evan. I knew that if Evan had been here, he would have already scoped out his place in the corner and planted himself. I would be the social butterfly talking and laughing with everyone. I would occasionally pop back over to see how Evan was doing. At that point, he would be having a good time with the guys.

    I was treading in new territory all by myself. All these functions were difficult. In the past, I always had Evan standing by my side. Us, like many other couples, had an escape plan, it was knowing who was going to throw up the white flag first! We always blamed the other for an early exit, Evan would be with his buddies saying, "Yeah, we have to get going, Mallory has to help her mom tonight." I could always count on Evan being the first to throw up the white flag to leave!

    After any event I was so emotionally exhausted from holding back my true feelings. My jaw would be so tight with tension from the fake smiles and stress I thought it would fall off my face. My back and neck were as stiff as a board. I would take a hot shower and lay on a heating pad for the rest of the evening. Everything that I wanted to say, and all the feelings I had, were buried deep inside. I would not allow any of them to see how utterly broken I was.

    The immediate change in our daily routine was anything but normal. The simplest thing would trigger my mind and throw my anxiety into overdrive. This was beginning to happen on a daily basis. The fear associated with the anxiety made me overthink everything. It typically was the worst-case scenario that something bad was going to happen.

I remember Bryan coming down with a cold, and instantly I was frozen with fear thinking he was going to die. I remember calling his pediatrician over the weekend, and the exchange answered. I thought I would hyperventilate hearing an unfamiliar voice. I screamed: "I want to speak with Dr. Balmerro, no, you cannot help me. My husband just died; I really need to speak with Dr. Balmerro!" The young lady on the phone was very compassionate but also very confused. "Miss, I am sorry, Dr. Balmerro is a Pediatrician, are you sure you have the correct number?" I responded tearfully," Yes, I am sorry, this is for my son Bryan. I recently lost my husband and, I don't know, dammit! Can you please page Dr. Balmerro."

Without hesitation, she told me she would attempt to reach Dr. Balmerro, and she did. Within half an hour, Dr. Balmerro called me back. I was blubbering uncontrollably while explaining that I had just lost my husband and that I did not trust anyone but him, "please help me Dr. Balmerro. I do not want Bryan to die!"

It took thirty minutes of being reassured over and over by Dr. Balmerro that Bryan was going to be okay. I had finally calmed down! Dr. Balmerro quickly made me feel at ease, "Mallory if it would make you feel better, bring Bryan into the office on Monday morning to be seen. It will be a quick in-and-out office visit. Mallory, are you sure everything is, okay?" "Yes, yes I'm fine Dr. Balmerro, I am just concerned with Bryan's cough, and after losing Evan I am afraid of losing him also." After talking with Dr. Balmerro, I went into the bathroom to pull myself together. That girl looking back at me from the mirror looked like an empty shell with eyes. A scared little girl looking for a closet she could hide in. I pressed a cold washcloth to my face hoping it would diminish the red blotches now covering my face.

I walked out to the living room to check on Bryan. He was in his normal position, sitting on the couch watching cartoons. "Hi, Mom. Who were you talking to?" "Oh, it was Hailey, she wanted to know what we were doing tonight for dinner." In my head I kept telling myself, "Be strong, and appear normal. Do not let your kids, or anyone else, see you like this, EVER!" I was concerned after getting off the phone with Dr. Balmerro, his question stuck in my mind, "Mallory, are you sure everything is, okay?"

If Bryan had only known the emotional and mental breakdown I just had, he would have known the one other important person in his world was close to losing it. I couldn't control my fear and anxiety, I felt at times that I was losing my mind. Nothing was minor and everything was magnified a thousand times. My heart was racing, and the tears would start flowing at any given moment. Dammit! Why can't I control this!

Well Monday arrived and I never did end up taking Bryan in to see Dr. Balmerro. He just had a cough and appeared to be doing fine. I was angry at myself for acting like a crazy, overprotective mother. Going off the rails over a simple cold just was not normal. I felt awful about interrupting Dr. Balmerro's weekend, crying like a lunatic, and telling him all our family's personal trauma. This was my young son's pediatrician. I'm surprised I didn't see Child Protective Services at my front door after that call!

What was I doing? I would tell myself over and over, "Mallory, watch yourself. Stay in control, they'll be coming for you with a straight jacket!" I honestly was not looking forward to seeing Dr. Balmerro at Bryans annual appointment. I did not want any pity. I was just humiliated by the way I handled the entire situation. I was weak. I needed to be strong again!

At times like this, I would get angry at Evan! He was not here when we needed him the most, especially when the kids were sick. Evan was always great with the kids whenever they got sick. Projectile puke, runny nose, fever, or whatever it was we were dealing with, Evan was a trooper. I felt that if Evan had been here, he would have been on the couch with Bryan lying next to him. They would be watching whatever cartoon or movie Bryan wanted to watch. Next to them, popsicle sticks stacked high on the stand, and the much-needed cup of Gatorade with a green straw hanging over the side. It was moments like this that you felt your family routine was hi-jacked that made you say, "When the fuck did our lives turn upside down? Where has the leader of this fortress went?"

Evan would have done anything for the kids, and the kids felt the same way about Evan. Every night I'd laugh at Evan as he came through the front door to our home. The barking of the dogs would be the evening announcement that he was home from work. As soon as Bryan heard that alarm sound, you could hear him bouncing down the hallway to see his dad.

Evan would flop down in his comfy recliner. Bryan at lightning speed would ambush him with a high-five, and the two of them would talk about their day. The moment always came when Evan would look at Bryan and say, "Hey, Bud, do you want to make some hard-earned cash?" Bryan would always answer with a sly smile, "Let me guess, Dad, you want me to take off your work-boots for 5 bucks!" I think this little routine had been going on since Bryan was big enough to lug those heavy work boots to the front door.

Watching Bryan struggle to undo the laces and get those heavy ankle-high work boots off every night made us laugh. Bryan would say "Come on, dad, at least pull your foot a little. Ewwww, these smell disgusting!" It was the ultimate challenge, but Bryan was being paid well, or so his dad thought.

Before Evan passed, a typical morning for the two of us had been waking up early, hopefully way before Bryan woke. We would sit at the kitchen table to have a cup of coffee and talk about all that was going on in our kids' lives or all the crazy shit that was going on in the world. Currently, the majority of the talk was about Hailey's wedding and Hailey graduating from college soon.

His little girl was getting married, and neither one of us could believe the time had arrived for her to even get married. One day you're watching them take their first steps and the next, you're walking them down the aisle. We had a lot of planning to do. It was going to be a beautiful wedding! Hailey and I would be running around checking out wedding venues, wedding dress boutiques, florists, DJs, and photographers. You name it, and it was on our list to see, hear, or taste.

I would drag myself into the house after one of these fun-filled days with Hailey, Evan would always look at us and joke, "It's beginning to look like I will have to buy a suit for this event, or can I just wear this?" Evan would point to his t-shirt and dark blue Dickie pants and laugh. Hailey would quickly respond, "Dad, a suit of course. I have wanted this my entire life! I promise I'll only torture you for one day." She was her dad's angel. She knew she had him wrapped right around her finger.

The stacks of papers, menus, and color options were beginning to take over my desk. Getting this all pulled together and organized was not going to be an easy task. Planning a wedding and college graduation at the same time had me running in a million different directions.

Evan left the planning up to Hailey and me. The cost was not going to be an issue for his only daughter's wedding day. He would give her the moon if he could reach it. There would be days he would say, "Mallory, instead of a big wedding don't you think Hailey would rather have the money to put down towards a home? The kids could have a small church wedding. This money would be a nice down payment for them." I could not wait to hear Evan present this to Hailey.

Hailey was not hearing it! It had been a dream of hers since she was a little girl, and now it was time for her dad to walk her down the aisle in a traditional church wedding. "Dad, I'll be graduating from college soon; I'll buy my own home. The only thing I really want is for you to walk me down the aisle!" That was it! The decision was made, and it was final, a big church wedding it would be!

As much as Evan hated the fact that he'd have to put aside his T-shirt and Dickies and don a suit for the wedding. One thing was certain. He was happy that this event would bring together a lot of the close family and friends that we had not seen in a long time. Since Evan's Dad had passed, we all cherished the opportunity to get together and see aunts, uncles, cousins, and close friends. We all certainly were not getting any younger.

After our morning coffee and idle chit-chat, the house would get a little livelier as Evan would intentionally stomp down the hallway, knowing it would wake Bryan. Without fail, Evan would give Bryan a little bear hug before he left for work, telling his Bud he loved him and would see him later. Evan's final stop would be the kitchen again, this time to fill his cup with the remaining coffee, give me a kiss and a hug, and off to work, he would go.

Today I look at that same coffeepot. It had been barely touched. You would never have seen that in our home prior to Evan's death. We would have had that finished off. Evan's favorite Dallas Cowboys coffee mug still sits in the same spot that it had been left, to the right of the coffeemaker, empty and waiting for him. I sit alone at the kitchen table. No conversations, no laughter, no stomping down the hall, or squeals of laughter from Bryan's room as Evan would rush through his bedroom door. Our home is now empty.

I am waiting, quietly praying to hear the slightest sound of Evan coming down the hallway. Pissed off, I grab the coffeepot and dump the remaining coffee down the drain. As I watch the coffee spill from the pot, I think, this is not the new normal I want. This new quiet in our home is unsettling. I feel it, and I know my kids feel it, also. Hell, even our dog knows that something is not right in this house. The glue that has held this entire family together for years is now gone. I must come to terms with all of this. I really don't have a choice in the matter.

I can recall the painful conversation I had with Hailey one morning. Hailey had seen me during my delusional daydreaming, which typically led me to believe there may be hope that I would see Evan walking down the hallway again. He will grab his coffee mug, smile at me, and sit down at the dining room table with me once again! Hailey knew that everything was not right with me. She would attempt to calm me down and say to me repeatedly, "Mom, it will never be like the normal we once had as a family, but a new normal for our family." Our first year without daddy will be filled with all new normals. It may not be what we are used to, and as painful as some things will be, we must try and push through this for our family."

I would nod my head in agreement with Hailey and thank her. For such a young lady she had so much wisdom and knowledge. As much as I knew what Hailey was saying was true, I did not look forward to this new normal or the pain that I knew would come along with accepting it.

What is a "new normal", and when will we see and feel this new normal in our lives? Does something instantly happen like magic, and then we feel normal? Do you wake up one day and that is the day that you actually want to leave the house and spend true quality time with people? Is this the time you become forthright with family and friends, no longer hiding all your pain and grief?

During this coming of a "new normal," I continued to keep my emotions buried, hidden far from my children. The smiling, positive character I displayed daily to the community only made me more angry and bitter. I was a ticking time bomb keeping everything bottled up inside. The cluster of unsettling emotions just ate at me daily, waiting for this new normal to occur.

THE DREADED FLU

Evan walked into the house, blurting out in disgust "Mallory, the doctor said it's the flu. Hopefully, you and the kids do not get it. It is draining the life out of me! This could not have come at the worst time; we are so busy at the office!" I looked over at Evan as he slumped in his recliner "Evan that sucks. I heard its going around. It's probably something you picked up at the office. The kids and I have been feeling fine." "Mallory, the doctor prescribed me some medicine for this cold. Would you mind running out and grabbing my scripts. I would really like to lie down and try to get some rest; my head is pounding." "Sure, I'll take Bryan so you can get some rest while we are gone."

I yell to our 10-year-old son, Bryan, "hey buddy, let's go, we have to go pick up daddy's medicine. He is not feeling well." My son Bryan, a soft-hearted, old soul, always so kind and caring, asked with concern, "What is wrong with daddy?" I look at Bryan and say, "It is just a really bad cold. His doctor said it's the flu. You really have no need to worry. Once dad starts taking his medicine, he will feel better in no time."

So off to the pharmacy, we go. As we walked in the door to the pharmacy, Bryan sighed heavily. He is looking directly at the pickup counter and the line is beyond long. I look at him and say, "Bryan that long line of people will move fast. We will be out of here soon. The pharmacies are always busy this time of the year. It's when a lot of people come down with the flu." I guess my explanation worked. Bryan heads off to explore while I wait in line for Evans scripts." A few moments later I see Bryan, his arms waving over his head, holding up a chocolate candy bar. He is trying his best to get my attention as I stand in the pharmacy checkout line. "Hey mom, mom, can we get this for dad, it's his favorite." How can I say no, the kid looks like he is running a triathlon trying to make it up to the counter. "Yes, Bryan, quickly bring it over so we don't hold up the line. I am sure that dad will be happy you bought him that candy bar today."

Finally, with the scripts in hand, Z-pack, Codeine, and the much-needed chocolate candy bar, we are headed out of the pharmacy! I looked over the information list attached to the scripts. They all look familiar to me; I know that I have been on these in the past. They always kicked in quick, and the recovery followed soon after. It will be smooth sailing for Evan once these get in his system!" I start the car up and we are off for home.

It certainly takes a lot to knock this guy off his feet, so for Evan to want to go to the doctors this morning he had to be feeling as sick as a dog. In all the years that I have known him, rarely did he ever take much time off from work for being sick. In late November, he had surgery on his foot to remove a large callous that made it uncomfortable to walk. There were times during his recovery his foot was painful and swelling. Evan always summed it up as just another Gout flareup.

During his recovery from foot surgery, he adorned a lovely black surgical boot and went into the office. I think he may have said that the worst part about it was taking all the jabs from the guys, "hey is that going to help your golf swing?", "Aww, you're limping like your favorite football player." Evan was a good sport and let it roll right off his shoulders.

Most of the employees that worked for Evan had been there from the time that they had gotten out of high school, to him they were family. I can remember Evan always pushing his employees to better themselves, helping them get their CDL or certifications for advanced training in the field. Evan never had that concern that if he gave them too much education that they would leave him for another job. It was important to Evan that he had trained skilled workers. He always felt it would benefit everyone overall. Evan had always said, it was important to have self-worth, having a skill or a trade meant you had a career for life, no matter where you traveled. I know so many of his employees respected him, he always wanted to see them all do well in life.

As I pulled into our driveway, I really could not remember the entire drive home from the pharmacy. It seemed like the car was on autopilot the entire way home. I often found myself lost in my thoughts while driving. I would arrive somewhere and wonder, "how the heck did I get here." Today, my mind was focused on Evan's health and getting back home with his medicine. If I knew Evan, he was driving himself crazy not being at the office today. I would not have been surprised if he had left for the office while I was gone.

I walked into our home and tried to make a small space on my dining room table to set down Evan's medicine. Bryan's Humpback Whale project for school was devouring my entire dining room table. There were endless pieces of ripped newspapers everywhere. The dining room table looked like Time Square after New Year's Eve with scattered paper everywhere! A bowl of sticky gook waiting for its next piece of paper, my favorite salad bowl covered in paper mâché currently shaped in the form of a whale's hump. I looked forward to the day of packing up this whale and sending if off to school with Bryan! I told myself, "Take a deep breath Mallory, it will all be back to normal in a week."

Evan was in the living room, lying back in his recliner. It appeared he had gotten some rest, but I could tell he was not comfortable at all. I made him a cup of hot tea with honey and brought it to him, quietly setting it down on the end table next to him. I don't know what it is, but it seems hot tea with honey is a magic remedy in helping to cure a cold. Growing up, every time someone was sick in our home, you would hear, "give them hot tea with honey. They'll feel better in the morning!" and here I am today, still following those old traditions.

I gently felt Evans forehead. He was warm, his fever was coming back, his eyes opened, and he looked at me. I handed Evan the hot tea along with his pills and said, "okay, let's get this medicine in you, so you start feeling better, and hopefully, tonight you can get some sleep." Evans hand trembled as he took the medicine from my hand. His eyes looked bloodshot from the lack of sleep. He looked at me with his tired eyes and said, "Thank you Mallory, I hope this does the trick, and Bryan thank you, buddy, for the candy bar. You're the best!"

Poor Evan, looked like complete hell. His body was feeling the full-blown effects of the flu. The hardest part would be keeping him home from the office so that his body would heal. If there was anything Evan hated, it was sitting idle. This guy felt that sitting in a doctor's office for a half hour to be seen was wasting his time. This was literally taking the time away from him getting things accomplished at his own office!

So often, when Evan was at a doctor's appointment, his phone would ring non-stop. He would get angry and frustrated and say, "screw it, I don't have time to wait here any longer!" Typically, it was an employee calling from our company just wanting to run something by Evan, or something had occurred at a site where they were working and wanted to keep Evan posted. I would get so frustrated and say, "leave your phone with one of the other office staff to manage it or shut it off!"

Often, the ringing did not stop, and Evan would get up and leave his appointment without being seen. As we walked out to the parking lot, we would argue, I would say "Evan, you have got to keep this doctor's appointment!" He would look at me and say, "My time is just as valuable as these doctors' time. Our company does not run itself. I have people depending on me!" and off he would go. I always felt defeated, but once Evan made up his mind, there was no changing it. He was as stubborn as ever.

Evan had been the man that wore many hats at the office. His favorite saying was, "The best helping hand is at the end of your wrist." When I look back, I don't believe there was anything in the early days of the business that Evan did not do. He basically was a one-man show with a few loyal employees. The company grew quickly, and Evan was attempting to control everything that came across his desk. I am sure that this got to be a bit overwhelming at times. We did eventually hire other office staff but letting go of that control was very difficult for Evan. Again, this man would be working

24-7. It never phased him. His drive to build a successful business was unwavering. In Evans mind, if his business were successful, it would benefit him, his family and all his employees. That is what drove this man!

If and when Evan would take a vacation with us, it would be someplace that was within driving range of the business. That typically meant, taking two vehicles in case Evan had to leave to oversee work related business. That did happen quite often. When we could break away, we would load the cars up at night and drive to Maine at 4:00 a.m. We would be racing down the Mass Turnpike, praying that Evans phone did not ring and ruin our plans. Although the kids were not big fans of that early start time, we always missed all the bumper-to-bumper traffic. The kids would smile as they were waking up to see that we had already made it to the beach. It seemed that once we were at the beach all the stress and anxiety left us, we could relax, dig our feet into the sand, close our eyes and just listen to the sounds of the ocean.

The get-togethers in Maine were some of our favorite vacation memories as a family. At times we would have close to twenty family members spontaneously taking the trip to Maine. We would have an enormous area encircled by beach chairs, coolers, and toys. The only thing missing was a family flag stuck in the sand, claiming this area as our own.

My husband was funny. He would show up on the beach wearing his knee-high black socks and white sneakers, after the family teasing commenced. He would always say "hey you never know when you're going to have to get up and drive back home. At least I'm prepared!" This would become a joke in the family that always reared its ugly head at family gatherings, "no white sneakers with black socks on the beach!" From that point on he would start bringing along to the beach, what the family would refer to as his Jesus sandals, his old worn-out leather sandals that he had for years.

Evan woke up from his short little catnap. It seemed as though he felt guilty that he had taken the time to rest. For some reason, this man always felt like he should be moving and being productive. Today he was not working at the office and felt that he really should be doing something other than sleeping. As soon as he would wake up, he would look at his phone to make sure there were no calls or texts that he may have missed. During the day, when he was awake, he continued to take calls from employees and customers. You could see that even these small efforts were draining him. He just did not have the energy to handle all these business calls. He was complaining that his head and back were killing him, and he was not able to get comfortable. I gave him more Motrin and fluids hoping it would alleviate his pain, but with the flu it was common to have all these symptoms.

 I walked into the kitchen to make lunch for Bryan and me. I yelled out to Evan, "Do you want anything to eat?" I had expected the response I got from him, "No, thank you. I really don't think that I can eat anything. I just do not have an appetite." Evan had barely eaten anything within the past 24 hours. I know taking that medication on an empty stomach would make him even more nauseous. I figured I would run out to the grocery store and pick up a few items that he might be able to eat.

 I looked at Bryan and asked him if he would mind staying home with his dad while I ran out to the grocery store. "Mom, of course not!" This kid was a homebody just like his dad was on the weekends. I went into the living room and looked at Evan, "I'm running out to the grocery store to pick up the ingredients for chicken noodle soup. Is there anything else that you want me to grab for you while I am out?" Evan looked at me, shook his head, and closed his eyes. I figured this would be an easy babysitting job for Bryan.

 Our ancestors had passed down all these homemade remedies. They must work, right? Weren't all these remedies a cure-all? Didn't all our grandmothers and our moms always give us chicken noodle soup when we weren't feeling well? Wasn't this a common thing? The hot tea with honey, the cold washcloth on our foreheads all these things were so comforting. Our old traditions taught us and set in our minds that this is what we use to help us feel better. I can remember my mom slathering us with Vicks whenever we had a cold. To this day, when I smell Vicks, it always brings me back to the day as a child when I was sick. I would be lying on the couch, the menthol smell, and the cold washcloth. We did not use strong medicine back then; it was always the basics.

    I pulled out of our driveway and rolled down my car window. The weather was unusually warm for April, it was in the high 70's, and here I am, headed to the store to buy all the makings for chicken noodle soup. I turned up the speaker volume on my car radio and noticed Christmas music was still playing. Wow, Christmas music in April! I liked the song that was playing, so I just kept listening to the station. I know it sounds strange, but Christmas music always comforted me. It brought back a lot of good memories. It gave me that sense of happiness, security, and reassurance, just like the holidays always gave to me with our family and friends gathered at our home.

    As I drove, I knew God was in control. I had this overwhelming feeling of calm and peacefulness. All was going to be okay. To reaffirm this, I said out loud, "Mallory, I know it may be a rough week, but we will get through it! Evan will be feeling well soon! That humpback whale will be off to school with Bryan, and life at home will be back to normal."

    I roll my shopping cart through the aisles grabbing anything that is related to "comfort healing foods," oranges, berries, nuts, some fresh leafy vegetables, a case of Ginger Ale, and let's grab these chocolate chip cookies for Bryan. I made my way up to the checkout counter and started plopping all the groceries onto the conveyor belt. The clerk looked at me, "looks like someone is going to be making chicken noodle soup, my favorite!", I responded, "yes, my husband has come down with the flu, and you know what they say about homemade chicken noodle soup.", she looks at me and smiled, "You bet I do! My grandma and my mom swore it was a cure all. Have a good day, honey, hope your husband feels better soon." I nodded and said a quick thank you and made my way back home.

I get home to find Bryan at the dining room table. He had been working on the paper mâché Humpback whale. I was impressed with his work for a ten-year-old. There in the center of the mess sits my favorite salad bowl, I see it coming in handy, supporting the large whale hump. The old wire hanger had turned out to make a nice swooping tail. Bryan asks, "What do you think, Mom?" as he grabs a chocolate chip cookie off the counter. "Hey, that's really starting to look like the Humpback whale that we read about in your book. I can't wait to see it once you paint it." "Yeah, it's going to look great, I can't wait to bring it to school!" I can hear the wheels spinning in Bryans head, as he rushes off to his room. "Mom, I'm going to make a boat out of Legos, and I'll add people also." I smile at Bryan; this kid's imagination never ends. "Mom, you know what else? It's going to be their mission to capture this ferocious Humpback whale!"

Legos, it seemed was a common interest for Evan and Bryan. They made a weekly trek to the store to see what Lego set they could buy. The more difficult and challenging, the better! As soon as Bryan would open that box, within hours he would have the latest and greatest Lego put together. Bryan was funny because he knew his dad enjoyed seeing all these sets put together and was amazed at such a young boys' accomplishments.

The trend continued, next Lego arriving home was the Lego Death Star, the mother of all Legos for this boy. Bryan worked with his dad on this for days, once complete the ceremonial unveiling and placement on top of his dresser. This went on with these two forever, it became a timed, creative challenge for them, Bryan always had to remind his dad "No Glue!" Evan had attempted the glue trick once and Bryan couldn't understand why his dad was using glue on his Legos "Dad, how am I going to use them again?" I guess in Evan's mind he felt that once the project was complete it was to live on for eternity in Bryan's room, but not the case in Bryans eyes!

"Evan, soups ready. Do you want to try and eat? You need a little substance in your stomach." As difficult as it seemed for him, Evan had a few spoonsful and handed the bowl back. "Mallory, I just can't eat. I feel like I'm going to throw up with just that little bit of food. I just don't have an appetite. I better just stick with Gatorade." I took the bowl back from him, I couldn't help but feel so bad for him. He couldn't tolerate food. The only thing he wanted was fluids, he had pain in every part of his body. I cursed the damn flu!

"Mallory, can you grab me some Motrin? I'm having bad back spasms. The pain is unbearable. I think if I lay down in bed, it may help." As Evan attempted to lift himself out of the chair, he moaned in pain. His arms were trembling supporting his weight. "Mallory, can you give me a hand, I don't have the strength to pull myself up." I ran over to Evan to help him. His body was like a ragdoll, and he had no strength or control of his limbs. I finally got him to our bedroom and helped him to bed. "Mallory, can you put the pillows under my back." Evan was restless, and I was doing everything I could to make him comfortable.

As the day went on it was apparent that Evan may need to go to the hospital, the pain in his back and head were getting worse. Evan's attempt at laying down in our bed was not helping his back at all. He was now asking if I would help him out to the dining room table. As I helped Evan out to the dining room table, I could feel his weight as I supported him down the hall. "Mallory, I just want to sit here for a while, I can't even turn my head, my neck is so sore." I ran over to the kitchen sink and got a warm washcloth and applied it to Evan's neck. Evan slid his arms out over the dining room table and laid his head down in the mess of newspaper scraps and paper. This is where Evan fell asleep. The sound was of a painful soft snore. His body was crashing. He was exhausted and in pain.

It was a Friday night, I knew I would have to make some phone calls and, hopefully, find someone that would stay with Bryan. I needed to get Evan to the hospital. I called Evan's sister Susan; she lives right down the road from us. "Susan, can you please come over and stay with Bryan? I have to get Evan to the hospital. Something is not right." It was not 10 minutes later, and Susan was at our house. As she walked into our house she said, "what is that smell?," I had started a steaming pot of Vic's on the stove, once again hoping it would help Evan. That plan and all the others had failed I knew he had to be seen by a doctor at the hospital. Susan looked over at Evan and agreed, he had to be taken to the emergency room, his color was off, and his eyes were bloodshot. I shuffled Evan out the door, trying to get out before Bryan caught us, I didn't want Bryan to see his dad so weak and sick.

I sent a quick text to Hailey to let her know that I was taking her dad into the hospital, I try not to alarm her by downplaying all my concerns. I think if I had called her, she would have immediately picked up on the fear in my voice. Evan was not doing well; I was on the brink of tears. I let Hailey know that I think it is best for her dad to go into the emergency room to be evaluated. I felt more than likely they would just give him some intravenous fluids and antibiotics. The prescribed medicine was just not helping him. Before I hung up, I told Hailey that I would touch base with her later that night or sometime the next morning and give her an update on her dads' prognosis.

As we walked out the front door of our home; Evan was insistent that he was okay to drive. "Mallory, I am okay to drive. If I am not driving, I'm not going!" I shake my head knowing if I argued with him, he would turn around and go back in the house. I walked with him to his side of the truck to make sure he is okay to get up into the truck. His hand grasping the strap and giving it all he's got to pull himself up into the driver's seat. It looked so painful to see him slouching to find a comfortable position to sit, his teeth clenched as he turned the truck ignition. I hopped up in the passenger seat of his enormous black truck, thankful at this point that he even agreed to go to the hospital. I don't even bring up the subject of letting me drive again, for him to agree to go to the hospital, he is definitely not feeling well!

As we are driving, I notice Evan is on, and off the shoulder of the road, I look over at him and ask, "Evan, are you sure you are okay to drive?" "Mallory, I am fine, it's these new tires on the truck. They are bigger and have a lot more tire tread. We are going to feel a little pull from them!" He is irritable, and I can hear it in his voice. The last thing I want to do is argue with him. I just tell myself to keep my mouth shut. He is the type that will turn around and say, "screw it," and go home.

We continue driving down the main highway he turns to me and ask, "where are we going?", I respond, "Evan, we are going to the hospital" he looks at me with the Deer in the headlights look, "oh, what's the best way to get there?" This man is looking at me with a confused look like I'm a hitchhiker he just picked up and is wondering where I want to go. I am now really scared, I feel my heart drop. This was so out of the norm for Evan. He knew this area like the back of his hand. These questions throw up a huge red flag that something is terribly wrong with him.

Evan has lived in this area his entire life, he has driven to this hospital several times, and is now struggling to remember how to get there. Holy fuck, what is going on here! I slide closer to Evan and keep my eyes on him the entire time. I am preparing to grab the steering wheel at any moment to keep us from crashing. Evan seemed as though he was in a trance. He may as well have had blinders on. He was driving as though his brain was on auto pilot. I kept making small talk, hoping it would keep him alert.

We are minutes away from the hospital, but I feel this ride has taken us hours to get there. I held my breath the entire way, praying we made it there safely. We gradually exit off the highway. Thank God we are seconds away now! Dammit, we hit a red light, and sitting there waiting for that light to turn green felt like an eternity! Finally, the light turns green, and we are still just sitting there, we are not moving. I look over at Evan, and he is sleeping at the wheel. At this point, I lose my shit; I'm crying and pleading with Evan to let me drive! "Mallory, I am okay to drive, look, the hospital is right there." "Evan, pull this goddamn truck over now!" "Mallory, I'm okay. I swear I'm okay to drive!"

We pull into the hospital entrance, grab our parking ticket, and try to find the nearest spot by the emergency room. I am so pissed at Evan right now, but my head is also spinning, wondering what in the hell is wrong with him. What in the hell was causing all this confusion? Was it the pounding headache? This kind of shit has never happened to Evan!

It is Friday, late noon, and the waiting room has a handful of people. I'm thinking this should be a fairly short wait to be seen. We go up to the registration desk and advise them of Evan's symptoms and tell them exactly what prescriptions he has recently been prescribed. The young lady at the front desk registration is very pleasant and assures us that someone will be right out to get Evan. It was no more than ten minutes; we have a wheelchair assist, and we were headed back to a room to be evaluated. In my mind, I think, all that Evan may need are intravenous fluids and possibly an overnight stay in the hospital. If all goes well, we will be home by midnight.

A young female doctor comes into Evan's room and begins to evaluate Evan, asking him several questions, "are you drinking are you urinating? How is your appetite? How long have you been running a fever?" I explain he has been dealing with the flu for the past week and the prescribed medications have not helped at all. The fever, back spasms, and stiff neck seemed to have gotten worse for him, almost intolerable. The doctor reassures us that with the flu, these are all common symptoms, sometimes, you bounce right back, and other times it just takes a little longer.

The doctor draws blood from Evans arm and sends it down to the lab. "Evan, we are going to start you on intravenous fluids and antibiotics. I think this may help with some of the flu symptoms you are dealing with. You should feel a noticeable improvement later tonight or in the morning." As soon as the nurse started the intravenous, I headed out of the room. I knew I had better call Hailey and let her know that we may end up being at the hospital all night. I did not want to leave the hospital until I knew the fluids and antibiotics were working; and Evan was feeling better.

I called Hailey's cell phone, and she immediately picked up, "How's dad feeling? I wanted to call you earlier. I just didn't want to interrupt the doctors or whatever may have been going on?" "Hailey, your dad is doing okay. The doctor drew some blood and is running some labs; they have started intravenous fluids and antibiotics as well. I think it may be a long night. Hailey, will you text your brother and see how he is doing? Please try to be very discreet about your dad, don't tell him too much." I knew if I called Bryan this late at night, it would just upset him. I also knew Bryan rarely answered his cell phone. In my plan of plans, Evan would be okay by morning, and we would be back home before Bryan even woke up.

Getting Bryan, a cell phone had always been Evan's idea. At the time, Bryan was only nine, and I just didn't think he was responsible enough to have one. "Mallory, come on all the kids have cell phones right now, what if something happens, wouldn't you want Bryan to be able to reach us?" "Evan, of course, I would want Bryan to be able to reach us. I also know that the first time Bryan lays that phone down at school or on the bus, it will be history!" A week later, after our conversation Bryan walked in with a Lego set in one hand and a cell phone in the other, "hey mom look dad bought me a cell phone, cool right?" "That's totally cool Bryan." So much for the let's wait until he is a little older and more responsible.

I knew as much as I hated to tell Hailey, I knew I had to tell her about the nightmare ride into the hospital with Evan that day. "Hailey, I'm going to need you and Noah to bring my car to the hospital and pick up daddy's truck. He can't drive. He fell asleep at a red light! I thought we were going to get into an accident or die on the way to the hospital today!" "Mom, is dad going to be, okay? What is going on with him?" "I don't know, Hailey; I just need you and Noah to please bring my car in before he is discharged." Poor Hailey, I had no answers for her. Maybe Evan was sleep deprived. Maybe the high fever was throwing off his judgement. I just didn't know. I wasn't going to chance it; he was in no condition to drive!

I slowly walked back to Evan's room; I could hear the sports channel coming from the television in his room. I walk in and find that Evan has fallen asleep. His 6'3" frame dangling over the edge of the bed, and an I'V tubing placed at the top of his hand, slowly dripping the much-needed fluids into his body. It gave me peace of mind, listening to the quiet rhythmic sounds of his breathing as he slept. I sat and watched him sleep for a while and thought. This is exactly what your body needs Evan. You need your body to rest and heal. I thanked God, over and over, that we were here at the hospital, and that Evan didn't put up a huge fight to get here. The ride in that would be something we would talk about at a later date, now, it's time for rest and healing.

"Mallory, let's get going. I'm feeling much better." I look over at Evan, he is sitting on the edge of the bed, raring to go, his color looking a little better. I guess I hadn't realized I had also drifted off to sleep. It was almost midnight; the day had taken a toll on both of us. I carefully unfold myself from the side chair that I had been sleeping in for the past few hours, "Well, Evan, you look much better! How are your headache and back spasms? "I think this is what I needed; I'm feeling a lot better." "Evan, if you're sure that you are up to leaving I'll go get the doctor; she will determine if you are going home tonight." Evan looked at me with that look, "Mallory, I'm going home!" I knew there was not a chance in hell at keeping this guy at the hospital. I had my fingers crossed as I left the room to go find the doctor, knowing full well that there was a 50/50 chance they would discharge Evan. I knew I was in for a fight if it was not what he wanted to hear.

I made my way to the nurse's station to see if the doctor was available to evaluate Evan for discharge. I waited out in the hallway until I saw the doctor approach Evan's room. I knew going back into that room, Evan would over-exaggerate and make it seem like he had been waiting a lifetime to get out of the hospital. "Good evening, Mr. Mills. I hear you are ready to leave the confines of this beautiful hospital?" As the young male doctor approached Evan, he quickly flipped through all the intake paperwork and quickly reviewed some information on his laptop. "It appears your blood work is not yet complete, but if you're feeling well, we will discharge you. If for any reason you are not feeling well after you leave, please get back into the hospital! We will contact you later today regarding your lab results. Also, I recommend that you schedule a follow-up with your primary doctor to be seen within the week. You are all set to go. Take care Mr. Mills." "Geez Mallory, I didn't think we were ever going to get out of there!"

The evening from hell was now over, Evan was feeling better, and we would be home before Bryan woke up. I helped Evan to his feet, and we headed out to the parking lot. "Mallory, where is my truck?" "Evan, I had Hailey drop off my car and bring your truck home. The ride in today was a little hairy, and I wasn't sure if you would be in any type of condition to drive home tonight." "Mallory, I'm fine, I could have drove!" As we got in my car, I looked over at Evan attempting to squeeze his large frame into my small sedan. This was not going to be easy. I know he was hating this entire situation, the small car, and my driving. Tough shit, I was driving!

    I realized as my stomach growled that neither of us had eaten since early yesterday, "Evan do you want me to stop and grab you a bagel and coffee?" "No, Mallory, I'm really not hungry, I just want to get home." This would be going on day three with barely any food for Evan, I'll chalk it up to the effects of the flu on his body. I'll try to get him to eat something later. For now, let's just get home!

    Rise and shine, its Saturday morning! I slept like shit; we did not get home until after 1:00 a.m. I am hoping that Evan was able to continue to sleep throughout the night. I got out of bed and head out to the kitchen to grab a cup of coffee and check on Evan. I looked in the living room, and Evan is laying back in the recliner. "Evan, did you get any rest last night? Are you feeling any better today?" Evan looked over at me, and I could tell by the bloodshot eyes that he did not have a good night. "Good morning, Mal, I slept okay. I just wish this damn headache and back spasms would go away. I'm going to go down to the office for a while and get caught up on some paperwork and phone calls." "Evan, please don't be down there all day. Your body may be on the way to recovery. I just wish you would take it easy once in a while." Evans comment back to me all the time, "Mallory, that business is not going to run itself!" As Evan walked out the door, I mumble under my breath, "I swear someday that place is going to be the death of you!"

    I decide while Evan was down at the office working, I would reach out to his primary doctor's office to discuss last night's events and my concerns. It is Saturday morning, and I knew I would get the exchange. I left a brief message and asked if someone would call me back as soon as possible. I did not want Evan to walk in and hear me on the phone with his doctor. He would immediately tell me it was not necessary.

My cell phone began to ring within 15 minutes after leaving my message with the exchange. "Hi Mallory, this is Penny calling back from Dr. Smith's office. I heard that you had to bring Evan into the Emergency room last night. What's going on?" "Hi, Penny. Thank you for calling me back so quickly. Yes, last night I did bring Evan into the Emergency room. They gave him intravenous fluids and antibiotics. They also drew some blood and submitted it to the lab. Penny, Evan has not been himself. The medication is not working, he is complaining of severe headaches, back spasms, and a stiff neck. Some of the things he is saying and doing are just not making sense." "Mallory, it may be the effects of the fevers and Codeine, is he taking the suggested Codeine dosage?" As far as I knew, Evan was taking exactly what it said on the Codeine bottle. By the end of the conversation, we both decided it would be best that Evan follow-up with their office on Monday morning.

Evan arrived back home after being at the office for an hour. I watched him as he walked into our home, his legs and back looked like they were made of rubber bands, he was using anything around him to support his body. "Oh my god, Evan, you have got to go lie down and rest. You can't keep pushing your body like this!" I took Evan's hand, "come on, go lay down and get some rest." I could tell by looking at Evan, he felt defeated, "Evan, this will all go away, you have the flu, and I can see it's kicking your butt. You have to stay home and get some rest. The office work is going to have to wait." "Mallory, I just don't know what is going on with me, I hurt everywhere. I can't focus or concentrate!"

With Evan headed off to our room to lie down, Hailey came barreling in the front door of our home. She looks at me with crazy eyes and says "Mom, have you been driving dad's truck, it is almost parked on our front patio." I look outside and sure enough there it is. The truck is up on our lawn, almost touching the patio! I immediately recollect my ride from hell with him as we drove to the hospital the other night, and know we have a serious problem! I take his truck keys from the counter, and I hide them. I know for a fact I'm going to end up in a screaming match, but he is not driving!

Evan wakes up a few hours later, complaining that his head is still pounding and his backpain is unbearable. I am alternating Motrin and Tylenol for the pain. I have dragged out the heating pad, ice pack, and anything else to help alleviate the pain. Evan is still not eating enough to even say that he has eaten. His stomach just cannot tolerate food right now, but he continues drinking fluids.

At 9:00 p.m. that night, we are all exhausted! Bryan is in bed; I'm lying in bed in our room and Evan has decided to stay in the living room in his recliner. I had set everything up on the stand next to his chair, drinks, medication, and tissues. At this point he can sleep wherever he wants, I just want him to be comfortable and out of pain. I'm glad that we will be going to see his primary physician tomorrow, hopefully they have a better idea of what is going on with Evan. We have exhausted all avenues in an attempt to get him feeling better. Was this really the flu?

I laid in bed thinking about how quickly things escalated in the past two weeks. This illness has really taken a hold of Evan and taken a toll on his body and was not letting up. It was just two weeks prior; that he was dragging me out to dinner for my birthday. He wasn't feeling that great but said he thought it was just a little cold and insisted that we go out." Mallory, you only turn 50 once, let's go celebrate!" "Ya know what Evan, you are right, let's do this!" This man never forgot a birthday or an Anniversary. As busy as his life was, he always carved out time for special moments, for the kids and me.

This whole "I'm taking you out to dinner to celebrate" turned out to be a surprise 50th birthday celebration for me. As we pulled into the local venue, I recognized all these cars. "Evan, what's Susan's car doing here, wait why is Noah's truck here? Evan is this what I think it is? I can't believe you didn't spill the beans about this!" For Evan to have kept this a secret was very impressive, he typically sang like a bird. "Did Bryan know about this, he was another one, just like his father, no secrets!" "He sure did, but I told him if he kept it a secret, he could get another Lego set! That kid could be bought!"

As I opened the door to the venue, I could see a walker setup right near the door for me. A huge banner hung on the wall with the words "Caution Senior Crossing." Bryan and his cousins were pointing at the walker and laughing. Bryan being the ambitious one dragged the walker over to me, "Mom, here this is for you to use today." Bryan ran away, laughing along with all our friends and family. "Thank you, Bryan, this old gal appreciates your kindness."

I looked at Evan, "How did you pull this together?" He smiled and said, "I was only the financier and driver. I was required to get you here without you finding out about it. Your sister Payton and friend Lexie made all the arrangements, the food, cake, and decoration's." I looked at Evan and gave him a kiss, "wow, this is unbelievable, everything looks great!"

It was fantastic seeing all our family and friends. We all chatted and caught up on everything going on in life and how we should all get together soon. I looked around the room. The kids were dancing as the D.J. played the music, and the atmosphere was perfect! Evan had picked out his place, laughing with the guys over in the corner. It was nice to see how much fun everyone was having. It seemed like it had been such a long time since we had gotten all together. I guess we all get wrapped up in life. The planning of Hailey's wedding and college graduation had kept us pretty busy this year.

A couple hours into the party I walked over to see how Evan was holding up. "Mallory, do you mind if I leave? I am feeling the effects of this cold. I'm going to try and sneak out. I'll have Brady drop me off at home." Evan rarely got sick, when he said he wasn't feeling well, he really wasn't feeling well. "Evan of course not, you should have told me earlier instead of trying to hang out here. Go home and rest, I'll see you in a couple of hours."

Brady is my older brother; he and Evan had always been close friends. The two of them were inseparable. It was a given during the summer months, every Sunday morning like clockwork, they would be off golfing. Later in the day, we would all ride up to Saratoga, stop for dinner then go watch our horse's race at the track. They could sit and talk about sports and old cars for hours on end. They had a great friendship! Today I was glad I could count on Brady to take Evan home. I know Brady, he is the caring type that is going to make sure Evan is comfortable before he leaves him. "Evan, do you need me to stop and get Motrin or Gatorade? Buddy, if you are going to need anything, let me know."

The party was wrapping up and I was looking forward to heading home to see how Evan was doing. I made a plate of food for Evan; I said all my "thank-yous" and goodbyes and out the door I went! The plate of food I had put together for Evan had such a variety; I was sure he would be tempted to try something. I know Bryan had a good time. He had made his own plate to go, which contained cupcakes and fruit. "Mom, were you surprised? Dad told me I better not tell you about the party, but I really wanted to!" "I was very surprised Bryan; it was a fantastic party! Also, thank you for not ruining the surprise. I heard you're getting a Lego set for keeping your lips sealed." Bryan looked at me and smiled.

For me, things had changed drastically in the last two weeks since then. The here and now of what I was dealing with frightened me to the core. It was time to stop reliving memories from the past. I had to go check on Evan. I wish I had magic powers or a special potion to make this all go away. I could not bear to see Evan in this much pain.

I opened our bedroom door; Evan is lying in bed with pillows piled high up behind him and throw pillows under his legs. As uncomfortable as it looked, I could tell he was sleeping, his soft snore every now and then filled the room. I quietly leave the room and find Bryan in the dining room working on his humpback whale assignment, "Mom, look at this, I did it! I made a boat out of Legos! I'm going to put it right next to the whale's tail, the whale is going to crush it with its tail!" "Bryan, wow, what a great job, wait until dad see's the finished product. You know he is going to be proud of the work you have done."

Sundays in our home was typically a quiet day, aside from the sound of sports blaring from the living room television. I would say that day was our day to rest and regroup as a family. Evan would be watching sports; I would be in the kitchen preparing dinner for our family night get-together. Bryan would be running around. He was always keeping himself busy, popping in the kitchen or living room throughout the day.

Today was nothing like our normal Sunday. Evan was sleeping in our bedroom, not in the living room watching sports in his recliner. Bryan had gone over to Colby's house to play. There was no sense in cooking a big meal when Evan had no appetite, I decided to cancel our family dinner that evening.

The quiet did not last for long, we had company non-stop, in and out to see how Evan was feeling. They all knew he had been in the emergency room the prior night and were all concerned for his well-being. It was odd today. The living room was quiet, with no football. I did not even turn the television on. My brain was on sensory overload, and the quiet was peace to my ears. Every time I have seen a family member pull up to our home, I would run to the door to avoid the doorbell ringing and the dog barking and waking up Evan. All and all, having a big family is great. Several of them dropped off more soup and cold remedies for Evan to try.

It seemed like all the company had finally dwindled, and it was so quiet you could hear a pin drop. The quietness was interrupted by my cell phone ringing. It was Lexie, "Mallory, hi, just checking to see if you were home. I will be dropping Bryan off in the next 10 or 15 minutes. The boys played great today, with no fighting at all! How is Evan feeling today?" I replied "He has been sleeping on and off all day. I hope his medication is finally kicking in. It's been rough for him these last few days. Lexie, thanks so much for having Bryan over. He needed to get out of the house for a while. I'll see you in a little while."

Colby and Bryan had been the best of friends since daycare. The boys were 2 and 3 when they met and from that time on, they had been joined at the hip. Throughout the years I had also become close friends with Lexie. We welcomed her into our home, she was like a sister to me. We did a lot together with the boys. It seemed one of us was always at the other house. The wine and the laughs always helped us when our boys played together. We had gone on several trips and outings together. We were always looking for something to keep these two energetic boys busy.

I see Lexie's car pull up. I ran to the door, again avoiding the doorbell barking dog alarm. I opened the door for Bryan, "hey buddy did you have a good time at Colby's house?" I could tell just by looking at Bryan he had a fun time. As Bryan ripped off his jacket smiling, he said, "Mom, we had so much fun. Do you think that Colby can spend the night tonight? We were making cool forts at his house but then I had to come home." The look on his face, boy oh boy you would think we just took all his toys away. "Bryan, we are going to have to plan the sleepover for another time. Right now, Dad is not feeling well." I was surprised at Bryans reaction, "Mom, you are right. I can have Colby over next weekend when dad's feeling better." Phew, that made it easy. I never thought I would hear that response.

I heard our bedroom door open; Evan was slowly making his way down the hallway. Bryan is super excited that his dad is awake. He cannot wait to show Evan what he has accomplished with his humpback whale assignment. I do not think Bryan gave Evan a moment to sit down and he was all over him. I laughed as I left the two of them to catch up. As I folded laundry in the other room, I could hear the excitement coming from Bryan and Evan, "Now Dad, remember this whale still needs to be painted then I'm going to add blue paper for the water, then I'm going to put the boat in near the whale's huge tail! Waammm the tail strikes!" All of this said with so much excitement and not one breath was taken between sentences! "Dad, do you think I should add anything else to it?" I hear them both laughing as Evan tells him, "Fill the whale's mouth up with all your Lego people, let them pile up, cascading out of the whale's mouth!" 'Dad, that's funny; I'll go find all my Lego people right now!" Oh boy, those two!

That evening as Bryan and I slept, I was woken by the sound of Evan's truck starting. I ran out to the living room to find Evan had left, how in the hell is he leaving, I hid the keys! In all the years that we had been married it was common for Evan to leave at odd hours for work emergencies. I instantly thought that something was going on at the office. It could be anything, like I said he would get calls all hours of the night for work related emergencies. I will text him in 20 minutes, which should give him enough time to get to the office and handle whatever the urgent matter is.

A half hour went by, and I messaged him, "Evan, is everything okay at the office?" Evans response sent a chill down my spine, "I drove to the hospital, I'm not feeling well, I think if they give me fluids again, I will be okay." "Evan, why didn't you wake me up, I could have had Susan stay with Bryan. You should not be at the hospital by yourself!" "Mallory, stay home with Bryan I'll be back in the morning." Grrrr, this man was as stubborn as ever!

I cannot fall back to sleep it's now close to 1:00 a.m. Bryan is sound asleep in his room. I keep telling myself to call Susan and just go to the hospital! I call Evan's phone, but he is not picking up! I send him a text about asking Susan to come over and stay with Bryan so that I can go into the hospital. We are going back and forth texting, when his final text comes thru, "Mallory, I don't need you to come into the hospital. They are giving me fluids again. Once they're done I'll be home. There is no need to wake Susan up. I'll be fine!"

Evan walked into our home around 6:30 a.m. looking just as exhausted as he did the day before. "Mallory, please don't ask me a lot of questions. I just want to lie down. I don't think the fluids helped; I still feel like shit! They did give me a different script to try, would you mind picking it up for me?" "Oh, Evan, I feel so bad for you. I wish there were more that the hospital could have done for you. I'll run out now and pick up the medicine." It was still early; I figured I would run out and get back before Bryan woke up.

Next week the kids had the entire week off for Spring break. I know Bryan is going to want to do something besides sit in the house every day. There was not too much I was going to be able to do with him since Evan was sick. I know one thing; he can use some of that time to finish that Humpback Whale project! The clutter on the table with Bryans stuff and the piles on the counter of Hailey's stuff was starting to make me anxious. Everything was lying around the house unfinished. Nothing was getting wrapped up! This flu thing with Evan was hanging on like the plague, it seemed like there was no solution or cure in sight!

I called Lexie as I drove to the pharmacy to see if she would be available to help with Bryan next week. "Of course, Mallory! We don't have anything going on next week. This will also give Colby someone to hang with." I was so glad I could count on Lexie; I had no idea what was in store with Evan's illness. I just wanted to make sure I had backup just in case I needed it.

When I picked up Evan's script, I noticed that it was to treat bacterial infections. How and where would Evan have gotten a bacterial infection? Was this something happening due to the flu? Could all of this somehow be related to his foot surgery? What in the hell was going on here? My brain was spinning, "no wonder all these scripts and hospital visits haven't helped. They've been treating Evan for the flu!

The first thing I did when I got home was find his hospital discharge paperwork. I needed to know why Evan was being treated for a bacterial infection. The blood work indicated a bacterial infection, they would like to do more bloodwork and run a few tests, blah, blah, blah. At the bottom of the discharge was Evans signature, along with the doctors. The notation read, "AMA-Against Medical Advice," are you fucking kidding me Evan!" I approached Evan and asked him what this all meant. Evan began to explain to me that the doctor wanted him to stay and be treated, "Mallory, there is no reason that they would have to keep me at that hospital! I can take these new pills here at home, they will do the same thing as those fluids they had pumping in my veins! I swore this man was going to be the death of me.

As the day progressed, things quickly declined! There was nothing I could do or give to Evan to control the pain he was in. He could barely get out of a chair, he was struggling, his arms were shaking, holding up his weight. His back pain was beyond manageable with Motrin. He was delusional about what he saw, and the random conversations were unreal. I would help him from his chair to our bed and 2 minutes later, he wanted to be back out in the living room. This would go on for twenty minutes, back and forth!

"Evan, sit down and watch television for a little while." I was hoping that the television would distract him so that he would be still for a few moments. Evan reclined back in his chair, as restless as ever. It looked like he was nodding off, one second, his eyes were closed and then suddenly open. He sat right up and reached for the remote control. He started flipping the channels and settled on a kid's cooking show. This seems odd to me. For as long as I've known Evan, it has been sports this and sports that, never a cooking show! If this is what he wants to watch then so be it, anything to settle his chaotic behavior. I walk out to the dining room and try to organize the mess of paper mâché lying all over my dining room table. I figured I could at least get this, and Hailey's paperwork organized while Evan rested.

The next comment I heard from Evan was oddly strange. "Mallory, do you think this Chinese food is making me sick?" I walked into the living room and looked at the television. The only thing I had seen on television was young kids at a cooking competition. I said, "Evan, what are you talking about? We haven't had Chinese food in over three months!" You're watching a children's cooking show! "Yes, but Mallory, do you think that food is making me sick." Holy Christ in heaven, I did not even know how to respond to him.

The day continued with Evan napping for short periods of time. This cycle goes on for most of the day. I feel awful for him. He is not able to get a solid hour's sleep. He is still complaining that his head, neck, and back are killing him. The spasms are sending shooting pain up and down his back. He is now feeling them in his legs. He is barely able to lift himself out of the chair without help. We are back to Motrin to alleviate the pain. I wish to God we had something stronger in this house!

I looked over at the stand near Evan and saw that his phone was vibrating. Unbeknownst to him, I had put his phone on vibrate an hour ago so that he could get some sleep. The ringing and the text messages never seemed to ever stop. I reached out to Evan's sister, "Sarah, I need you or one of the guys to stop up here and get Evan's phone. He is trying to sleep, and that thing keeps ringing! I also don't think he is in any condition to be handling business calls." I brought Sarah up to speed on Evan's morning so that she understood what I was dealing with at home.

As I waited for Sarah to arrive at our house, Evan looked at me and said, "Mallory, I think if we go back to that hotel with the waterbed, I'll be able to sleep. I really think it will help my back." I did not respond this time, and I knew the expression on my face was meaningless to him. I felt my heart sinking, my concern for him and what may be causing these irrational statements had my mind in a tailspin. We have never been to a hotel with a waterbed! When we moved into our first apartment, we had a waterbed, but that is about it. Hell, that was over 20 years ago!

My mind is in overdrive. I'm thinking of anyone and everyone that I can call to help me! I look over at Evan. He is struggling to get out of his chair again. There is very little strength in his legs to support his body. I help him to his feet; this time, he tells me that he wants to take a shower. For the love of God, give me strength to help this man. A shower now, why? "Evan, sit down on our bed. I'll get the shower ready for you." How in the hell am I going to manage this by myself?

I quickly call Hailey and tell her I need her to come over now! Her dad has been acting strange all afternoon. I am hopeful that Hailey can convince him to go to the hospital. When Hailey arrives, Noah is right behind her, thank God! Maybe one of them can talk some sense into this man and get him to go to the hospital. "Mom, where is dad, why are your clothes wet?" "Hailey, your father insisted he needed to take a shower! He was adamant that he was fine on his own, but obviously he wasn't! He has been moody and delusional all day. He is not listening to a word I say to him!"

I picked up my phone to call my neighbor Lexie to ask if she would keep an eye on Bryan, "Lexie, can you come over and pick Bryan up soon? I don't want him to see his dad like this. I have to get Evan to the emergency room!" It broke my heart to have Bryan see all this happening today. "Mallory, I'll be over there as quickly as possible!" I went back to my bedroom. I had gotten Evan out of the shower earlier and he was still sitting on the bed. I helped Evan get dressed and slipped on his sneakers.

I called for Bryan to let him know he was going over to Colby's house. "Bryan, get your things together, Lexie will be here soon. You're going to be having dinner with them tonight. I have to run dad out to his doctor's appointment." I could hear Bryan down the hallway, "Woo-hoo! Hey dad, I'm going over to Colby's house." Evan walked down the hallway with Bryan and gave him a hug. "I'll see you later dad, I hope you're feeling better soon."

I started to think again about Penny's comment about the Codeine. Was it possible that Evan was over-medicating himself? I went over to our kitchen counter and picked up the bottle of Codeine cough syrup. There really was not that much missing from the bottle, so maybe it was the fever. I could not figure out what was making Evan act and talk the way he was. I just kept praying he would be back to the Evan I always knew and loved.

It took us over an hour to convince Evan to go to the hospital. I am glad that Noah and Hailey were there to hear and see the way that Evan was acting. At one point, he was asking if the outfit he was wearing was okay to wear to the hospital. Never in my life have I ever seen Evan worried about what he was wearing! Evan was such a humble man; he was never out to impress anyone. This man was satisfied with dickies, and a blue T-shirt every day!

Noah helped Evan into his truck. He seemed so weak, he struggled to pull himself up into the truck. Noah gave Evan a final push up and he got him settled in the front seat. Evan was a little lopsided, but he was at least finally in! I climbed in right behind them and from the backseat I was pulling and trying to get Evan so that he was in an upright position. Not a peep from Evan about driving, he sat quietly in the passenger seat. Hailey was behind us in my car as we headed to the hospital. All attempts at calling an ambulance were out the window, there was no way I was going to get this stubborn man to go in an ambulance. I was just thankful we could get him to go at all.

As we drove to the hospital, Evan seemed to be talking about anything and everything. Some of the conversations made total sense, and some of it was clear out of left field. Evan wanted to talk about anything, just not going to the hospital! Noah kept the conversation going, even if at times, it did not make any sense to him. Noah got a complete review of the new tires that Evan had just put on his truck, as well as a lengthy conversation about his favorite Cowboys football team. Evan talked about playing football with his brothers when he was younger. It seemed like Evan just wanted to drive and talk that night, nothing else.

With the hospital in sight, I felt so relieved Evan would now get the care he needed.

THE MAKING OF A MAN

The prior day as I drove home from the pharmacy with Evan's script, I recall looking over at Bryan. I thought about how fortunate we were to have him in our lives. We thought for the longest time that we could not have another child. We had been trying for years, and nothing! Evan and I came to a point where we just said. It's in god's hands now. If we are to be blessed with another child, then it will happen. We have to stop stressing and beating ourselves up over it.

So, it was to be. Almost 13 years later, we were blessed to find out we were expecting a second child. We were ecstatic and completely over the moon with the news and couldn't wait to tell Hailey. Let's just say that having this conversation with our 13-year-old daughter did not go the way we had planned. "Mom, what? You're going to have a baby, you're 38 years old, and you're not walking in my school looking like that!" This conversation may have gone over better if the timeline were closer to her being in the 5- 8-year age range. She would be 14 years old when the baby was born, a whole new generation starting.

Hailey did eventually come around as we began to write down baby names, "wouldn't it be awesome if it's a boy and we can name him after papa Earl!" Hailey loved her papa. She always talked about him. He was so patient and loving with all his grandchildren. He would sit outside under the big old Oak tree and watch his grandchildren play for hours.

Papa Earl had planted that Oak tree in the family yard 50 years ago. It was one of the favorite places for the grandkids to play. Hailey felt in her heart that her papa had planted it purposely for his grandchildren to enjoy someday. That old Oak tree had been a gathering place for the young and old for so many seasons. It provided shade from the hot summer's days, displayed some of the most brilliant-colored leaves in the fall, and was the absolute best climbing tree all year round!

We couldn't wait to tell Evan's mom that we were expecting. As soon as the words rolled out of Evans mouth, I could hear her screaming with streaks of joy, "oh my lord, we have a baby on the way!" With the passing of Evans dad, 3 years prior, in 2001, the vail of darkness felt like it may be beginning to lift for the family. Finally, after so many years of trying to get pregnant we looked at this new birth as a blessing from above. We looked forward to our next OBGYN appointment so that we could find out the sex of our child. We were both hoping that it would be a boy, to carry on Evans father's namesake.

A few moments out in the waiting room seemed like a lifetime, and then "Mr. and Mrs. Mills, the doctor will see you now." As we sat in the doctor's office, we could see the manila envelope, just sitting on the doctor's desk, holding our child's gender. I think you could have heard a pin drop, as the doctor was opening the envelope in slow motion, I was screaming in my head "hurry up dammit". The doctor looked at us over his glasses and said, "It appears you are going to have a baby boy." Evan looked at him and, said, "Did you just say baby boy?" Evan's look was that of someone that had just won the lottery. "Yes, you are having a baby boy!" Holy hell those were the words we wanted to hear. I know Evan was in his glory and certainly Hailey would be happy to hear that we would be using papa Earl's name.

When Evan called his mom the second time it was to tell her we were having a baby boy, this time we put her on speaker phone. I could hear her crying and thanking the lord and yelling "Earl, we have a baby boy on the way, bless you Lord for this gift." See, this little man that would be coming into the world in 7 months would be the first baby to carry on the family namesake. This was going to be a big pair of shoes for Bryan Earl to fill. This was a moment our family had been praying for, for years.

To look back when Evan's father passed, our family's lives changed tremendously. Earl was like that one strong brick holding up the front porch from crumbling, once that one strong brick was removed the smaller pieces began to crumble to the ground.

Eventually that front porch, which was once the gathering place, was no longer there. The one individual that had brought soundness and strength to the family was gone, his years of hard work and devotion to his family were over, and it was now his time to rest.

For Evan, losing his father changed him completely. Evan was always a hard worker but now, there was no looking back, he had his nose to the grindstone 24-7. In Evans eyes he must now fill the role of his father, to be there for his mother and eight siblings. He would be the one to handle any issues that may arise in the family, and to make sure this tight knit family stayed together. This is a role that would consume his life, but in his eyes, it did not matter, this is what his father would have wanted for the family.

The days in the office would get so busy for Evan that he would forget to stop for lunch, but he made it a point to check in on his mom every day, no matter what! Evan knew from the time his dad had passed that his mom would not worry about any finances, no bill would be left unpaid, no home repairs would be left undone. His life plate was on the verge of overflowing, and it did not matter to Evan, he would make it work, even if it meant working even harder!

The bond that Evan had with his father was unexplainable, it was as if the two were a mirror image, walking, talking, just about everything in life, they shared the same exact core values. As a young man, Evan worked alongside his dad in the family business. It was not an easy job and living in the Northeast with the line of work that they were in. You had to be able to tolerate the high temperatures in the summer, and the frigid cold days in the winter. Evan would work 7 days a week to ensure that he was taking the brunt of the work so that his dad did not have to work so hard.

As his dad got older and was no longer able to drive, they would take off for drives, sometimes leading them to Maine to enjoy lunch at one of their favorite restaurants and a quick stop at the Seabrook racetrack. There was nothing Evan wouldn't have done for his dad. Their passion and enjoyment in the horse racing world, led us to purchase our own racehorses. The summer trips with family up to

Saratoga, watching the horse's race, and the exuberant amount of energy laughing, eating, and enjoying each other's company was amazing. These are memories, our family will treasure forever, the pictures on our walls will tell a story to our children, and grandchildren for years to come. The moments I got to spend with papa Earl are memories I will cherish forever.

Being part of Evan's large family was always exciting, something was always going on, baby showers, birthday parties, kid sleepovers, we had an abundance of kids, so the fun never ended. I think one of our favorites, was our Sunday family picnics at Evans parents' house, a small corner lot on a dead-end street. To me this felt like the perfect place to raise their large family. We all brought a dish to share, the same thing each weekend, with time the recipes got even better. The pool would be open, you could hear the kids, splashing, laughing, and screaming. The younger children would be nearby in the sandbox, digging roads and building castles. Nearby, you would find a small wooden swing, slightly moving in the breeze. On these warm summer days, you would find many of the adults taking shelter here under the shade of that tall Oak tree.

Early in our relationship, I always thought Evans family could be compared to those mushy family shows that aired during the holidays or the television series that had all the children, and everyone got along great! The mom would stay home, make dinner, and at night, you would have shared stories about your day. The end of the night would bring kisses on the forehead, with each sibling showing love and respect for one other. This is exactly how I had always felt since meeting Evan and his family. The polar opposite of how I was raised, always feeling emotionally detached. I felt so fortunate to have met Evan and given a chance at a beautiful life like he had always known.

Evan was one of nine, he had 4 sisters and 4 brothers, all of them felt like they grew up with a best friend to play with. I remember the first time going to Evan's house, it was Christmas, that overwhelming feeling of "will I fit in, will his sisters like me?" Will his parents approve of me! I had such a great time that evening, there was nothing I wanted more than to be a part of that family.

I do not think it was even a year later when Evan asked me to marry him, I knew the moment I met him I wanted to be with this man for the rest of my life. I can remember that day like it was yesterday. I was the designated babysitter for my younger cousins, as most of my family attended a friend's wedding. Evan showed up at my house, as I was attempting to get the laundry done, the kids were running around screaming and cartoons blaring from the television. Evan pulled me aside and said, "Mallory, I want this someday, all of this, with you! Will you marry me?" With unfolded clothes hanging over my arms, I did not hesitate to answer, "Yes of course I will!" This was one of the happiest days of my life!

From that point on every holiday, we were jammed packed in Evan's childhood home, wall to wall with adults and kids talking, laughing, and having a great time. Evan's mom, Ruth, was such an amazing baker. She would have been in the kitchen for days before a holiday preparing homemade pies and cakes from scratch, which would have put the best chefs to shame. Ruth was old school, nothing was bought and made from a box, and she knew every trick to make the best desserts by scratch. I smile now, remembering how throughout the year, she would save old Folgers coffee cans. At Thanksgiving she would fill those cans with all the ingredients for Pumpkin bread and bake them in her oven. I would walk into her house and see each Pumpkin bread neatly wrapped up in Reynolds wrap, all ready for each of us to take home. Ruth's homemade baked Pumpkin bread was undeniably the best Pumpkin bread, I had ever had!

I always looked forward to the holidays at Ruth's house, the aroma of the Turkey Roasting, or ham baking, the 10-gallon pan of homemade mashed potatoes. My father in-law Earl was always in the kitchen helping Ruth pull together these out-of-this-world meals for the family. All the aromas hit you as soon as you opened the front door. Ruth and Earl appeared to make this all seem so easy, always pulling off such a huge family meal without a hitch. I guess the years of raising a large family kept the process moving like a well-oiled machine.

We are very fortunate that Hailey picked up on all her grandmother's baking skills, from the homemade pie crust, zucchini, and pumpkin breads. This was a sweet memory for us during the holidays. The aromas now coming from our own kitchen brought us back to such a beautiful time in our lives. Thanks to Hailey's grandma Ruth, I know that someday, Hailey's children and grandchildren will experience some of the best times in the kitchen, followed by some of the best desserts!

My mother-in-law Ruth did not skip a beat when it came to the holidays. She would buy for every one of her children and all her grandchildren. To watch Ruth at Christmas, you knew that her pride and joy was right there in her living room, she cherished every moment. Ruth would talk about the Christmas holiday and how her and Earl would be up until 2 a.m. trying to get all the final gifts wrapped and placed under the tree. They would finally get to bed and find 3 or 4 of the kids standing by their bed at 5 a.m., gently tapping them to inform them that Santa had arrived.

I was in awe of Ruth and Earl, their patience and love, they not only showed to their kids, but all their grandchildren, and they had a lot of them. These were the moments that you just wanted to keep in your mind forever. It did not ever matter what they were doing, watching television in their recliners or drying dishes in the kitchen. They would hop in a chair to read a book to one of the kids, push them for hours on the swing or hold them and rock them. I could now see why Evan turned out to be the man that he was, a kind, loving, gentle giant to everyone. I do not believe I had ever seen any of the kids leave their parents' house without giving them a hug and a kiss on the cheek. This family was about love, caring and being there for one another, and I was so happy that I was now a part of it!

There was one Christmas Eve, I don't think any of the kids will ever forget. Evan had this brilliant idea to climb a tree at the neighbor's house and place a battery-operated Christmas bulb on one of the tree limbs. Evan casually walked back into the house and nudged me, "Mallory, look at the tree over there." I looked out the window and seen this red glow flashing high up in the tree. "Evan, the kids are going to be so excited!" We sat down at the kitchen table as though nothing was going on and waited for one of the kids to spot the red flashing light.

As the adults sat at the table the kids would come out to grab a cookie or drink from the kitchen, not noticing a thing. This continued for 15 minutes before one of them spotted the red flashing light. It was three words that were said that drew 12 small children to the kitchen window, "I see Rudolph!" With eyes as big as saucers they pointed out the window, "hurry, hurry, its Rudolph. He is flying over the house next door!" Every kid in that house was plastered to the kitchen window screaming, "look, look, I see Rudolph, Santa is coming!".

Evan stood over in the corner, smiling as he watched how excited the kids were. His mom and dad were laughing at the kids and all their happy excitement. I think this may have been one of the easiest nights; we got the kids loaded in the car and home early from my in-laws. All those little faces that had been plastered to the window are now adults. They still talk about that night they seen Santa and Rudolph flying over the neighbor's house.

As all good things must come to an end, after the passing of Evan's father, we sold all the racehorses. Evan no longer had the desire to own them. His passion for the horse races was something he shared with his dad, and now it was a sad, painful reminder that he was gone. The Sunday gatherings for picnics slowly dwindled the holiday gatherings began to shift out to other family homes. It was as though the light from a slow-flickering candle had finally gone out. A large gray cloud had suddenly engulfed this family and sucked all the happiness out along with it. It hurt seeing this happening to the family. All the traditions for so many years that kept this family together were unraveling like tattered strings.

I vowed to Evan that I would continue the big family holidays in our home!

WE ARE NOT DEALING WITH THE FLU!

I walked into the emergency room with Evan. In my hand I tightly clutched his medical discharge paperwork. As I'm filling out the emergency intake paperwork, I see Evan looking at me. He is waving me over, "Mallory, I need to go outside to get some fresh air, I feel like I'm going to pass out." I grab Evan's arm and quickly escort him out to the sidewalk. As we are standing there, he says, "Mallory, I think you should go back inside and get someone, I don't feel right, I need to sit down."

I looked at Evan. He appeared sweaty. His hands were clammy. I am thinking that at any moment this 6'3" guy was going to come tumbling down on me, and there would be nothing I could physically do about it. Evan is over a foot taller than me and built like a football linebacker. As Evan leans on me, I am using all my strength to pull him next to the building. I could feel the dampness in the shirt he was wearing. It was late April; you could see the perspiration rapidly evaporating from his skin.

The walk to the wall seemed to have taken us hours to get there. I breathed a sigh of relief as I gently guided Evan down the wall where he could sit on the concrete window edge. "Evan, are you okay? I'm going to leave you here for just a second. I've got to get help." I ran back into the emergency room screaming, "Help me, there is something wrong with my husband. Someone, please go out there. I don't know what is wrong with him!" I am screaming this over and over, as I try to find a wheelchair or anything that I can bring to Evan, this man is ill, sitting outside in 30-degree weather! Someone fucking help me!

It was not long before two nurses approached me, and we rushed out the door to find Evan still slumped along the wall. Evan looked as though he was struggling to stay upright, his arm pressed against the concrete window frame, shaking to support himself. My heart was breaking at this moment, a man so big and so strong was so helpless. The medical team quickly got Evan to his feet and settled him into a wheelchair. Evan's skin looked pale and pasty, his lips dry and cracked.

The medical staff proceeded to whisk Evan into the nearest intake room of the emergency room. The nurses in the room with us began to ask Evan questions about his symptoms. I could see that Evan was having a tough time recollecting events over the past few days. I finally had to interject that Evan was just here 24 hours ago. I handed the discharge paperwork from the prior night to the nurse. She proceeded to bring up Evans electronic medical record. I said, "I have no idea what is going on with him, he was diagnosed over a week ago with the flu, he is not getting any better with the Zpack prescribed to him, and this discharge paperwork mentions something about a bacterial infection. Does he have Meningitis, what is it?" "Mrs. Mills, I'm going to get the ER doctor. We need to review Evan's medical record. Right now, I need to get an I.V. started on your husband. He needs fluids asap. A tech will be in here shortly to place the I.V."

The nurse left the room, and a young medical student arrived a short time later. I noticed as he entered the room, he was already wearing purple latex gloves, as his hand pushed the door. I see him reach for Evan's arm and I yell, "What are you doing? You just opened that door with those gloves on, and now you think you are touching my husband!" What in the hell was this kid doing, Evan was already dealing with some form of a bacterial infection! The young medical student proceeded to open an alcohol swap packet. He looked at me with the alcohol wipe waving in his hand and says, "No, I am going to wipe down my gloves with this alcohol wipe. It will sterilize my gloves." As he begins to proceed wiping down his latex gloves, I walk over to him and say, "You are not touching my husband until you remove those gloves and put on a new pair!" The student looked at me completely in shock, like who am I to question him? I looked at him again, "Don't touch him until you remove those gloves dammit!" He looks at me as though I'm wasting his time, how dare I ask such a thing!

You would have thought I had just disciplined a small child as he huffed and puffed ripping off the soiled gloves and proceeded to put new ones on. I thought I was going to lose my shit at that moment! I had worked as a medical office manager for over 8 years, and I thought, what in the hell was he trying to pull? How many other times has he pulled this shit and gotten away with it!

After the soiled purple latex-gloved medical student left the room, the nurse returned. "Evan, we are going to be moving you to your own room. We are going to start stronger intravenous antibiotics to rid you of whatever is wreaking havoc on your body. Whatever this infection is, it has been resistant to all the other antibiotics we have given you. We are going to run some more blood work. This time we are going to test for Meningitis. This bacterium tends to be one of the bacteria that at times is resistant to certain antibiotics. Fingers crossed that today, we find the culprit behind all your symptoms. Mrs. Mills, we ask that you wear a mask until we have gotten the results back and have a better idea of what we are dealing with." I am now feeling hopeful that Evan is going to get a thorough work up. To know that we are now moving in a direction that could have Evan healed and back to normal was music to my ears.

I watched as they rolled Evan out of the room. I had made up my mind that this time I was not letting him leave this hospital until he walked out of this place feeling 100% better! There will be no, "Mallory, let's go I am feeling so much better." No, not this time! I know how Evan is. He would say to me all the time, "Mallory, I don't have time to sit here. You don't realize how much I have to do at the office." Evan always pushed himself. He never listened to his body. He was a strong tough, stubborn man, and nothing was going to sidetrack him!

I was finally allowed to enter Evan's room. It was an incredible sight to see. I could not believe the number of tubes with fluids pumping into his body. I could tell that Evan was already irritated and did not want to be there. He turned on the television and started watching the sports channel. I looked over at him, which at this point he had all his attention focused on the television. "Evan, are you feeling any better?" Evan turned toward me and said, "Mallory, no, I don't feel any better. I'm giving this an hour and I am leaving!" Oh, my god, here we go again. I knew this was not going to be easy. To sit here and try to explain to Evan that his health is much more important than that business, is like talking to the wall! I figured it would be best if I left the room to give each of us a little space before it ended in an argument.

With Evan distracted by the sports channel I figured I would go to the cafeteria and grab us coffees. I needed a little away time from him so that I could update the family on what little information I had at the time. Honestly, I really had no update for them, we had been at the hospital for hours and they continued to slowly rule out the cause of Evan's illness. I know that Hailey and Sarah would be waiting for me to give them a call. I knew with Hailey's college schedule she could either be in a class or she could be doing clinical rotations I figured I'd hold off and give her a call later when I had a better understanding of what was going on with her dad. Sarah on the other hand had been holding down the fort at the business. I wanted to touch base with her and let her know that we were still status quo on what was going on with Evan.

I called Sarah and she answered immediately, "Mallory, how is Evan?" "Sarah, he is doing okay, a little grumpy that he must be here, but he is not leaving this time! They have him back on intravenous fluids and strong antibiotics; they are testing him for Meningitis. Whatever he has is resistant to all the antibiotics that have been given to him." "Mallory, let Evan know that everything at the office is fine, I don't want him worrying about this place. We all just want him to get better! If you need anything or if you have any new updates, please call me." "Sarah, I'll give you a call later once the other blood results come back. I'm hoping that the next blood results will tell us something. Thanks for everything." With the murky coffee water in hand, I walked back to Evan's room, praying that this time there would be an update.

Not even five seconds after entering Evan's room, "Mallory, where have you been? I haven't seen a doctor or nurse come in here for at least an hour." I started to purse my lips together. "Mallory, I don't want to hear it, I'm not staying here any longer!" I wanted to respond that I had not even been gone an hour so that was entirely impossible, but at that precise moment the doctor walked into Evan's room. "Mr. Mills, hi, I'm Dr. Pitier. First off, I want to let you know the results for Meningitis have come back negative. We are also waiting on a couple more blood results to come back. What we would like to do at this time is a CT of your head. We would like to see if there is anything contributing to these headaches that you are having." I did not even want to look at Evan at this point. I held my breath and waited for his response, what I heard could have floored me! "Of course, Dr Pitier, I'm just as curious to find out what is going on with me." I looked at Evan, and silently thought, I'm sorry but did an alien just take over this man's body, he has been fighting me ever since we left our driveway!

As they wheeled Evan down for his CT scan, I thought that we were starting to make some progress. Who knows one or two nights in the hospital on aggressive antibiotics would be exactly what Evan needed. I know for a fact it was going to be difficult to even keep him here overnight. The way Evan responded to the doctor made it appear that he was now on board to find out exactly what was going on in his body. I was trying to figure out exactly how long we had been dealing with this. My dates were getting all jumbled together, I think we were going on a week and a half with this and no positive improvement.

It was an hour later before I saw them wheeling Evan back down to his hospital room. He seemed even further agitated that he was still here in this hospital and all he wanted to do was go home. "Mallory this is beyond ridiculous I do not know what is taking them so freaking long to figure out what's going on with me! This is bullshit!" "Evan, we have to find out the results of your CT scan I really think it's best that we spend the night here in the hospital." Mallory, they don't even have a neurologist here today to read my CT scan. They are out of their mind if they think I'm staying here more than one night!" "Evan, I think you are exhausted, hungry, and on top of that, you have been sick for days. It's been a long day for both of us, I'll go down to the cafeteria and grab us coffee and some soup." "Mallory I'm fine I don't need anything I just want to get the hell out of here!" I figured before this escalated any further, I would give each of us a little breathing room.

I only took enough time to run down to the cafeteria and grab a couple bottles of water and I went back to Evans room. I walked in the room and noticed he was opening and slamming the drawers on the side table. "Mallory, where in the hell is my cell phone?" "Evan, I gave your cell phone to Sarah earlier today, she is handling everything at the office. I spoke with her earlier and everything's going fine. You are in no position to handle business matters right now; you need to focus on your health and getting better." At this point Evan was pissed, his heart monitor was going off. I swore at this point he was going to have a heart attack! "Mallory, I want my phone!" "Evan I'll call Sarah; I'll have her bring your cell phone into the hospital if that will make you feel better. Please just lie down and rest for now."

The emergency room nurse came in to check Evan's vitals, his heart rate was still high. Evan was tossing and turning in the hospital bed, his body was too long for the bed, his legs were hanging over the foot board. There was no way for him to get comfortable. I asked the nurse before she left if they had any recliner chairs that Evan could sit in so that he would be comfortable. The nurse brought back a recliner chair. Evan attempted to get comfortable in it. The damn thing was so small Evan looked like a giant sitting in it. This chair is made for an average size person! Evan would go from the chair to the bed and back to the chair, he was up, and he was down. Over and over, I would stand up and grab him, I was so afraid that he was going to fall. He seemed so dizzy, confused, and disoriented. I would plead with him, "Evan please sit down and try to relax we will be out of here soon." That was a lie, we were not going anywhere!

Once again Evan got up and this time, he said he was leaving. This man could barely stand on his own. He was swaying back and forth; the I.V. lines had reached the maximum extent they could go. "Evan, you must sit down! You are going to rip out your I.V. lines, dammit!" With all my strength, I started pulling him back onto the bed. He fell back on top of me. I rolled him over on his side so that I could get up. I kept telling him over and over again that he was staying, "God dammit Evan, we are not leaving until we have a diagnosis on what is going on and how to treat it!"

At this point I was just telling Evan anything he wanted to hear. I was trying to calm him down, nothing was working. I was getting so frustrated one minute I'm saying we'll be leaving soon. The next I'm telling him to sit down. I needed to speak to a nurse, Evan's temper was flaring, he was mad as hell, but his body was like a jelly fish. All that pent up energy was turning to anger. I was having a hard time taking care of him in this condition. I pressed the call button to signal for help.

I was standing near him next to the bed. He was sliding his body to the side of the bed again. I was afraid he was going to land on his ass on the floor. I grabbed his arm to pull him back onto the bed. At one point, Evan lost his temper and said, "if you take my arm again and tell me to sit down, I'll fucking kill you!" As he tried to stand up, he fell into the side dresser, almost falling over. The next minute he would be sitting down like nothing had happened. Never in the 29 years that I knew this man had he never been violent or verbally abusive, something was going on in this man's brain! A nurse arrived in the room, I told her that Evan needed something to calm his nerves, he was acting like a caged animal.

As the hours passed, Evan began to get even more delusional, he looked at the privacy curtains in the room and asked, "Mallory, why are there boards on the windows? You should take them down. It's so dark in here." He would ramble on about calling people back about scheduled jobs. One of the men had been dead for over a year. He would start conversations with ghost, "I am going to need a dump truck and trailer on that job." That was how it had been going for the past hour, sporadic crazy conversations. Evan continued to try and get up, saying, "Okay, Mallory, I'm going to head into the office now." This was making no sense to me. What in the hell were they pumping into this man?

Evan was in no condition to walk. He was so weak and delirious that he didn't even know what he was doing or saying. I kept pressing the call button, and the response for assistance was slow or not at all. I could not keep a nurse in the room with me. At one point, Evan got up again, unraveled the dressing holding his I.V., and started walking towards the door. I jumped up from the side of the bed and grabbed him at the waist and pulled him back onto the bed. I was having a hard time controlling Evan. I was exhausted and he was out of his mind.

Before Evan tried to get up and walk again, I ran to the hallway screaming, "Can someone please help me? I can't manage him by myself I need help!" A nurse came in to help me. Evan was half on and half off the bed. The nurse went out to the hallway and called for another nurse to help her get Evan moved back onto the bed. I watched as both nurses attempt to get Evan back up on the bed. I see them struggling to get his 6'3" frame positioned on the bed without falling off again.

Once they have Evan back in bed, I noticed the other nurse was focusing her attention on the I.V. and the gauze dangling down from Evan's hand. Evan has attempted to rip this off so many times it looks like hundreds of threads are hanging down off his hand. The nurse begins to take the same gauze and wrap it around Evan's hand and takes a piece of sterile tape to secure it back on his hand. I look at the nurse in disgust and say, "Why are you doing that? I can't even believe you're not putting new gauze on him!" She looked at me as though I was stealing her precious time. She begins to unravel the old gauze and replaces it with new gauze and sterile tape. I know they think that I'm the biggest pain in the ass, but I didn't care! This is my husband, and he was going to be given the best care!

It was late in the evening, and I wasn't sure how much longer I could handle Evan by myself. I called Evan's sister Sarah, "I need you to come to the hospital I can't do this alone I need help!" It was not even 20 minutes later, and Sarah walked into Evan's room. I was so relieved to have someone there to help me. Together Sarah and I struggled with Evan, getting off the bed and helping him back onto the bed. His legs were over the footboard at the end of the bed, his frame was hanging way over, and he kept shifting his legs to the side, which would cause him to start sliding off the bed once again. This went on for close to an hour. The nurse came in and removed the footboard, which finally helped. It got to a point where it seemed like the nursing staff was fed up with our constant need for assistance with Evan.

I was aggravated, I was exhausted, and I was worried about my husband. I wanted Evan out of this hospital tonight! Sarah agreed to stay in the room with Evan, as I located the nurse manager in the ER. I told her I wanted my husband transferred out of here immediately. I felt the level of care he required could not be met in this hospital. I rattled off all my concerns that we had experienced the entire evening dealing with Evan, the lack of nursing support the lack of compassion. I wasn't blaming it on anybody I just expected so much more. For the hospital staff not to show compassion to Evan, it was breaking my heart. What happens to the people that come to the hospital that don't have family or close friends with them, what kind of care do they get?

The ER nurse was apologetic and said she would speak to the ER doctor about transferring Evan. Within 15 minutes, the ER doctor was in Evans room asking why I wanted him transferred. I recapped the last 3 hours and said I felt it would be in Evans best interest to be transferred to a hospital fully staffed that can handle his needs. I could tell that the ER doctor was not happy, almost offended about my request to transfer Evan. I know he thought that I felt his hospital was falling short in providing a higher level of care to Evan. After three hours of this bullshit, I really did not care how he felt, my main concern was Evan!

I waited in the room with Sarah, hoping that one of the larger area hospitals would accept Evans transfer. An hour had passed, the ER nurse manager came to Evan's room to advise me that the two local hospitals were not able to take a transfer that evening. The hospital had decided it would be best to move Evan to a patient room up in ICU. He would begin to receive one-on-one care from here on out, until he was transferred out to another hospital. The thought of moving Evan to the ICU made me feel a little better. I would continue to pray that Evan improved, and we could get him transferred the following day.

At this point Evan was not talking only moaning, it was a moan that you would hear if someone was in a lot of pain. He was no longer attempting to move. His heart rate began to increase, and his vitals were not looking good. I would look into his eyes, and it just seemed like two empty holes with no one there. They assured me moving Evan to ICU would be better, he would be monitored closely by the doctors caring for him. They wheeled Evan out of the ER and took him to the elevator for his transfer to ICU.

Sarah and I arrived in ICU, we could see the doctors in the room with Evan. One of the physicians came out and said that they would need to intubate Evan and put him in an induced coma. Evan's heart was not doing well, and they felt there was too much strain on his heart with everything going on. Sarah and I were asked to wait outside his room until they had intubated Evan. I looked over at Sarah, her eyes are red and swollen, tears still streaming down her face, just this whole thing has turned into our worst nightmare. We are both feeling helpless, not knowing what direction this will all go in.

As we waited in the hallway, I noticed a female walking down the hallway toward Evan's room. She was wearing hospital scrubs and carrying a sealed bag of tubes and other medical equipment. I was assuming all of this was for Evan since she had opened the door that adjoined his room. It was a small room that appeared to be a sterile washroom, with a stainless-steel counter and sink. Above the sink the wall contained latex gloves, a soap dispenser, and some paper towels. I am watching her through the glass door as she opens the bag. She is oblivious that I am there. I see her take the contents of the plastic bag that she had just carried in and dump them on the stainless-steel counter.

This is the same exact area I had just seen the doctors washing their hands prior to entering Evans room! I can still see drops of water on the stainless-steel counter from the doctors that had just washed their hands! I swung open the door and screamed, "you are not putting any of that in my husband. None of it is sterile at this point. You never washed your hands after opening this door, you didn't even bother to put on latex gloves prior to removing any of that equipment, you carelessly just threw them on an un-sanitized counter!" I could see the doctors in Evan's room, turn their heads in our direction to see what the commotion was. She looked at me as if to say "how dare you tell me how to do my job! She did not say a word to me. She quickly scrambled to pick up everything off the counter. Once she had all the tubes together, she looked at me and threw everything in the trash bin outside the door and stormed away. If my eyes were lasers, I would have pierced a thousand holes through her body! I did not take my eyes off that lousy piece of shit until she turned the corner at the end of the hallway. I just could not believe the lack of safety and hygiene I was seeing in this hospital; it was like no one was required to follow any fucking protocols!

    I sat back down next to Sarah, "Is this the kind of shit that happens in the ICU? My husband is critically ill with a bacterial infection and, "Ms. I can't wash my hands does not even give two shits about him. What in the hell is going on here!" Moments later the same woman returns, she does not even look in my direction. This time she brings the bag directly into the ICU room where the doctors are waiting, the curtains are drawn, and we wait.

    After a 45-minute wait, we were allowed to enter Evans room, Evan had more wires and tubes hooked up to him, and machines around him were beeping as they kept track of his vitals. I can't help but to look at him and cry, saying over and over again, "this was never the flu." This man that I've spent close to 29 years with, lying here helpless. A tube was down his throat to help him breathe and in an induced coma. How did we go from the flu to this? It was all unimaginable.

    I reached for Evan's hand and swore I was not leaving his side; I was going to make sure that they were giving him the best care. I would often think back to the days when his dad was getting older and would tell his kids "When it's my time, I don't want to be in a hospital, I want to be home with my family, don't ever put me in the hospital when I become ill!" I would fight and possibly end up in jail before I left this man's side! I prayed so much throughout that night, saying "please Lord do not let this be Evan's time. He is far too young and has so much to live for."

    The male ICU nurse on duty was very attentive and caring to Evan. He was thorough in his explanation so that we understood exactly what he was doing and why he needed to do this for Evan. He explained at this time they were getting his heart stabilized and monitoring the infection as well as giving him as many intravenous antibiotics as his body could handle. I appreciated everything that he was doing for Evan. As the evening hours dragged on it was clear to me that this nurse loved his job in the ICU. My only wish is that we could have had him stay with Evan for his entire stay at the hospital.

    It was early morning, and the shift was changing, and a new ICU nurse would be taking over soon. The caring and compassionate nurse from the prior evening said that Evan was beginning to spike a fever, it was currently 101. He told me we should not be concerned; Evan would be closely monitored in the ICU and treated as needed. The nurse taking over the morning shift arrived. I watched her for a moment, washing her hands, putting on her latex gloves, attentive and listening to the other nurse that would soon be off his shift. I prayed hard that she would be as good as the young gentleman from the prior evening. We would have to wait and see.

    During the change of shift, we are asked to leave Evan's room so that the new shift nurse was brought up to speed on Evan. Sarah and I took this opportunity to go downstairs to the cafeteria and grab a cup of coffee. I don't think either one of us had slept at all in the last 24 hours, our bodies were running on caffeine and high anxiety. My mind kept rehashing all the events that had occurred in the last two weeks. I couldn't figure out at what point all of this just got the hell out of control! I knew I had to touch base with Hailey and let her know how her dad was doing, I dreaded calling her with no good news. I also had to touch base with Lexie, Susan had said she dropped Bryan off last night to spend the night with Colby. I figured it was best that Bryan was spending time with Colby and keeping his mind occupied.

I called Hailey and gave her an update on her dad, she said she would be coming in after her class to see him. I called my good friend and neighbor Lexie to find out how Bryan was doing, he of course was doing great with Colby, playing, and watching movies together. I was a little more forthright with Lexie on Evan's condition. I was not sure how long I would need her to watch Bryan and I wanted her to understand the severity of Evan's condition. Lexi was crying at the other end of the phone and told me not to worry about anything, that Bryan could stay with them as long as needed.

As Sarah and I waited in the waiting room, the Neurologist arrived. He said that they wanted to take Evan down for a Lumbar Puncture to withdraw some cerebrospinal fluid, I had to sign off on the consent form to perform the procedure. I didn't care how many procedures they did if it was going to help Evan get healthy again! I wanted Evan to be walking out of that hospital by the end of the week. We had now been in this hospital for two days, all the blood work, and intravenous antibiotics, and still nothing seemed to be working!

I walked back to Evan's room with the Neurologist, another Dr. was kneeling by Evans feet, examining them. As she looked at Evan's feet and his legs, she took a moment to look at me and explain, "Mrs. Mills, I'm Dr. Wonnsock with Epidemiology. I am noticing in my examination of your husband that his bacterial infection may have come from the recent surgery on his foot. I don't want to alarm you, but the black spots on his foot may be an indication that clotting has led to a stroke. We are going to bring Evan down for another CT scan, as well as a Lumbar Puncture. This will help us better understand what we are dealing with. Once we complete these tests we can sit down and discuss things further."

My head was spinning, a stroke, at what point did Evan have a stroke? Was this the reason why he was acting so strangely and saying the oddest things to me? "God, please tell me this is not the case!" As Evans stretcher was wheeled out of the room, all my composure I had been holding together just slipped, the tears just started like a dam had broken loose. For the past two weeks we had been doing everything in our power to get Evan the best care, for what we thought was the Flu.

I walked back to the waiting room. Sarah saw the tears in my eyes, "Mallory, what is going on, what did the doctors say?" It was between sobs, I told Sarah everything the doctors had said about Evan. I immediately called Hailey; I really needed her here at the hospital. I was reluctant about how much information I wanted to share with Hailey over the phone. I felt it would be best if she just came to the hospital and we both sat down with the doctors together.

I didn't know the extent of the damage from the stroke, I honestly wasn't sure if Evan was ever going to talk again. This would crush Evan if he was unable to run his business and physically be involved in the day-to-day work. I'm not sure if sitting in the office all day would satisfy Evan! I know this man; he will push himself and be back on his feet in no time. When he sets his mind to something, it gets done, there is no stopping him! I know there will be a lot of rehabilitation, but we will get through this together.

Hailey arrived with Noah; we waited out in the waiting area for Evan to return to his room in the ICU. I told Hailey as much as I could but asked her to save some of her questions for the doctors. I could not bear to be the one delivering this information to my daughter, I knew when she heard it directly from the doctors it would break her heart. Since Hailey and Noah had arrived, Sarah decided she would go into the office for a while. All our employees had been calling and no one knew what was going on with Evan. Sarah wanted to make sure she sat down with all of them face to face to let them know how Evan was doing.

After two hours the Neurologist came to the waiting area, he said that Evan had a bacterial infection raging throughout his body, they were doing everything they could do, to manage the infection and his high fever. The more information that I received from the doctors, the less hopeful I became about Evans progress. Hailey was anxious to see her father, she did not want to believe anything the doctor had just told us.

When we returned to Evan's room, he was alone, the nurse was not in the room. Evan's right arm was positioned slightly under his back his right hand wedged between the bed and his hip. When they performed the lumbar puncture and returned him on his back, they did not notice they lodged his arm and hand beneath him. I honestly could not believe the shit I was seeing! Mother fuckers!

Hailey was looking at his vitals and noticed his temperature was at 105. Hailey and Noah went into the washroom and started wetting down paper towels with cold water and applying them to Evan. I raced out to the nurse's station. The ICU nurse in charge of Evan was sitting at the nurse's station, I looked at her and said, "Why isn't anyone managing Evan's fever it's up to 105. His arm is wedged beneath him, does anybody in this friggen place care!!!" The Neurologist I had just met with was sitting at the desk. He looked at the nurse and advised her to administer medication immediately and properly position him in bed. All the way back to Evans room I was mumbling out loud, I don't even know what I was saying I was just so pissed off at the staff!

Evans room was hot, with all the machines running in the room it had to have increased the temperature by 20 degrees. The air conditioning was barely keeping it below 70 degrees. We were doing everything we could do to cool down Evan's body temperature. At one point the nurse said, "If you continue to wet him down, you're going to give him bedsores." "We're not "wetting" him down, we're applying a cold compress to his body, so it cools down, his temp is 105 degrees. If someone had monitored his temperature, we wouldn't have to do this!!" I knew my dialogue with this nurse from here on out was going to be strained.

I proceeded to ask the nurse if they would put a fan in Evan's room to help cool it down, and her response was, "We don't have fans in the hospital." I was losing my patience with this hospital. The lack of hygiene protocols, the lack of compassion shown to Evan were wearing on my last nerve. I wanted Evan out of this hospital, and I wanted him out now! I walked out of Evans room and proceeded to walk over to the nursing station and asked for the nurse manager on the floor. Come hell or high water I was going to wait here all night if I had to. I was going to speak with the nurse manager and get Evan out of this fucking shithole of a hospital!

"Hi, Mrs. Mills. I'm Karen Wells, the ICU nurse manager." "Ms. Wells, the prior evening I requested to have my husband Evan transferred out of this hospital. This hospital cannot accommodate the care that he needs! I want to know what is going on with the transfer request. I want to know why the nurse managing Evans care left him in his room with a temperature of 105 degrees. I want to know why I can't have a fan in Evans room. That room has got to be close to 80 degrees! I have also witnessed staff at the hospital not following safety or hygiene protocols!" I laid it all out! I told myself "Mallory, not one tear, you better be strong for Evan and make this happen!"

Ms. Wells looked at me empathetically and said, "I understand Mrs. Mills, we are working with a local hospital to get Evan transferred this evening, I'll keep you posted on the progress. I am sure we can find a fan to put in your husband's room, give me a little while to track one down. Later this evening, I will speak with the ICU nurse handling Evan's care. I'm sorry you've had to deal with all of this at our hospital."

As the evening wore on Evan's fever slightly improved, and miraculously a fan appeared in his room. The temperature decreased slightly with the fan in Evan's room, at least now it didn't feel like a hot sauna. I saw a new doctor come into Evan's room; like a hawk I was all over him. My trust in anyone at this hospital was now gone. I hadn't slept in 48 hours and the adrenaline was pumping through my veins! I was now the "Gate Keeper." No one was going to touch Evan unless I knew what was going on first!

He was a young doctor, and he introduced himself, "Mrs. Mills, hi, I'm Dr. Krelin. I will be handling Evan's care until he is transferred out later this evening. I looked at him and asked, "Which hospital and what doctors will be managing Evan's care, once he is transferred out?" "Mrs. Mills, I will confirm that information with the staff here, once I know I will get back to you." "Dr. Krelin, what is the status of Evans condition? Does the other hospital feel that they can treat and manage the bacterial infection?" Mrs. Mills, we are transferring Evan out because we feel the other hospital will have more resources available in providing the care Evan needs right now."

"Dr. Krelin, is that it? Is that your answer? You can't tell me either way right now if Evan is going to be, okay?" It was so frustrating. There were so many vague answers coming from him. "Dr. Krelin, are you from this area? Are you familiar with the specialist at the other hospital? Do you know their names?" The way Dr. Krelin hesitated on his answers led me to ask him, "Are you a Locum Tenen? Are you filling in on an as-needed basis for this hospital?" Dr. Krelin responded exactly as I had thought, "Yes, I am a Locum Tenen. I am very familiar with this hospital; I've worked here on and off for the past year."

Dammit, I immediately knew that he was a Locum Tenen, a temporary doctor filling the needs of the hospital! I did not know this doctor; I did not know his specialty. I just knew that Evan was a very sick man, and we had just spent two days in this hospital, still not having a definite answer on his care going forward. So many red flags had gone up. I still strongly felt that if I had gotten Evan transferred out sooner, he would still have had a good chance at beating this!

I waited in Evan's room with Hailey and Noah. We were all praying that the transfer would happen soon. The temperature in the room felt like a hot muggy night in July. The fan was barely providing any circulation in the room. The nurse kept the sliding glass doors to his room open due to the heat. Poor Evan, you could see the sweat dripping down his forehead. To keep him cool we would grab a cold washcloth and apply it to his forehead. I just waited for the nurse to tell us again that we were going to give him bedsores, dampening him down like this. The guy was friggen roasting in this room!

As we continued taking turns rotating out the washcloth for Evan, the Nurse "We have no fans at the hospital," came into Evans room and said they were preparing to transfer him out. This was the best news I had heard all day, finally we are going to a facility that could manage his care. Thank you, lord! As I left the room, I felt a spring in my step, thinking we still had a chance! I watched as the ambulance crew came in to move Evan out. I touched Evan's hand and told him how much I loved him and said, "hang in there. I'll be right there with you through all of this."

I waited outside the elevator until I was 100% positive that they had Evan, and that he was getting out of the hospital! The ambulance crew slowly guided the stretcher onto the elevator with the I.V. pole, and all the tubes hanging off from Evan. I looked at this man that only a week ago could have taken on the world. One of the strongest, smartest, and kindest men I'd ever met in my life, now dependent on all these doctors and nurses. Not one of these people knew Evan's story, nor did they have the time to care about the type of human being he was. If only they knew the generous, caring man that he was, maybe his life would have meant so much more to them.

I got into my car for the first time in days, we were finally leaving this hospital! Hailey and Noah were right behind me in their car, all of us following the ambulance to the hospital. It was also the first time I had been alone in days, I prayed out loud to God, "Please let this man live. He is a good man and deserves to live." I silently mouthed the words over and over, "Evan please hang in there. You will be at the hospital soon." The ambulance with its lights and siren blaring finally pulled into the emergency room entrance. I pulled around to the visitor's parking garage with Hailey and Noah pulling up alongside of me. Thankfully, we found a parking spot on the ground floor; it was so late at night there were hardly any cars in the parking garage. I breathed a sigh of relief! I was happy that I had Hailey and Noah with me for support, I did not want to do this alone. We grabbed what we needed and raced into the hospital to track down Evan.

The automatic doors to the hospital slide open. I felt a little calmer, like I made the right decision to move Evan, to escalate his care to a skilled hospital. All the fighting, crying, and arguing with staff at the other hospital drained me, I can now focus on Evan at this hospital. I was a little more familiar with this hospital, both of our children were born here, it was one of the leading hospitals for patient care in the area. "Okay, Mallory, get your bearings together, Evan is where he needs to be now. They will take good care of him," I told myself this repeatedly as we walked through the hospital.

I approached the front desk information booth and inquired if Evan had been placed in a room yet. The young man directed us to the ICU waiting area, where a doctor would come and get us once Evan was settled in. The waiting drove me crazy, all the worst thoughts went through my head, "what if Evan didn't survive the ambulance ride here", what was taking them so long? As we waited Evan's, nephew Jake arrived. Jake and Evan were extremely close, Evan was like a father to his nephew Jake. Evan played an important role in Jakes life and helped him through so many obstacles in life. To see them together was like watching a comedy routine, the best sense of humor, always making everyone around them laugh. This was the same nephew that had us all laughing so hard at the beach our drinks were shooting out of our nostrils. Evan always said, the best vacations in Maine had been when Jake and his family joined us.

Jake walked up to us and asked, "How's he doing?' I looked up at Jake and said "We haven't been able to see him yet. It's been over an hour since he arrived" Jake sat down beside us, put his head in his hands, "I can't believe this is happening, why him, how?' There was just no explanation for it, I had no words to explain what happened to Evan. We had all just hung out the week prior at my surprise 50th birthday party, how quickly things had changed within that time.

"Mrs. Mills, good evening, I'm doctor Stelar, we have moved Evan to a room. I want to let you know during the ambulance transfer here Evan went into AFIB, and we had to stabilize him. When you go to his room you will see that we have him on a mechanical ventilator. I can take you to his room now." My poor Evan was doing everything in his power to fight for his life, AFIB, which is Atrial fibrillation is a common type of irregular heartbeat. Evans body was testing him with everything it had, but Evan was not having it. He was a fighter!

    Dr. Stelar directed us to the room that Evan was in. It was a large room. The Mechanical Ventilator attached to Evan's face appeared to be so tight and painful, but I knew this was keeping him alive. He looked comfortable in his bed, with no feet hanging over the footboard this time! The room temperature was cool, and in the corner was a single chair. Evan's room was directly across from the nurse's station, giving me a sense of calm, knowing that someone always would have an eye on him. "We are going to keep your husband stabile this evening, in the morning Neurology will do some more tests on him." I walked over to the small chair in the corner and sat down. It was so quiet in the room; I watched as Evan slept. The monitors registering every heartbeat. The tubes feeding fluids and antibiotics into Evan's body seemed to be coming from everywhere. I sat down in the chair listening to the slow rhythmic beep, beep, echoing in my head.

    Noah, Jake, and Hailey all stood near Evan's bed, not saying a word, just looking at him as though they could not believe that this man in the bed was Evan. I could hear them talking about our trips to the beach, and all the good times that we've had over the years. The BBQs at each other's house, and the near burning down of our home when the grill caught on fire. They avoided any conversation related to Evan's current condition; it was right in our faces. It was something we did not want to acknowledge. We wanted to remember the good memories of Evan. Jake could always tell a story that would make Evan laugh so hard he had tears rolling down his face. I was hoping that Evan could hear them talking and in his own way smile.

    I must have fallen asleep in the small chair in Evan's room. I couldn't even recall the last time I had slept; I didn't even know what day it was. The ICU nurse was gently tapping me on the shoulder, "Mrs. Mills, I'd like you to go home and get some rest. We will take good care of your husband here in the ICU. We don't need you running yourself down. Physically and mentally." I quickly responded "No, I'm not leaving Evan, he needs me here!" Hailey, Jake, and Noah, reiterated what the nurse had said, "go home, get some rest, we will stay here tonight, if anything happens, we will call you right away." As much as I opposed the idea of leaving Evan, Hailey said "come on mom, I'll walk out with you. Jake and Noah will stay with dad tonight, we both need to get some rest and be here for dad in the morning." I walked over to Evan's bedside, stroked his hair, and told him how much I loved him; I did not want this to be the last time I saw him alive; I told him to keep holding on for me.

When I arrived home, it was so dark, quiet, and depressing. Bryan was now at my sister in-law, Susan's house, Lexie felt the boys need a little break from each other. I really missed him and just wanted to give him a hug. The phone calls to him had been quick, I did not want to give him too much information about his dad, only saying that he was still sick. I lay in bed tossing and turning just thinking about Evan all night, praying for a miracle to happen.

Beep, beep, beep, my alarm was going off and for a moment I thought I was back in the hospital with Evan, and the heart monitor was going off. I was half dreaming and half awake, I jumped in the shower and quickly got dressed. I wanted to be at the hospital to talk with the doctors to find out what was the next step with Evan. I grabbed my toothbrush and thought, this is the first time in three days, I've brushed my teeth, showered, or even combed my hair. The dark circles under my eyes showed that my body was dragging to keep up. I didn't care, I was going to push myself and do everything I could until Evan was back home with us again.

SILENCE & SOLITUDE

As I walked in the hospital, I appreciated the fact that it felt like there was life here. The sun was shining, and people were smiling. I could hear soft music playing, people were in and out of the gift shop with flowers and balloons. It all put me in a very upbeat positive mood about meeting with Evan's doctors. I walked in Evan's room. Noah and Jake were still holding down the fort, I couldn't thank them enough for staying with Evan the prior evening. Jake and Noah both looked at me, both talking at the same time, "I think Evan is improving, he was moving his feet last night!" I looked at them, smiling, "Oh my God, I prayed all night hoping to see some improvement in Evan" We were all smiles, this was a good thing, this could mean so much for Evan's recovery. Noah and Jake gathered up their coats and headed out the door as I waited for the doctors to make their rounds. I thought, if love could keep this man alive, he would live forever, and this may be just what is happening. I couldn't wait to share with his doctor what Noah and Jake had just told me.

"Mrs. Mills, Good morning, I'm Dr. Sastoraki, I'm going to take a look at Evan and check his vitals and see how he is doing." I walked along with Dr. Sastoraki over to Evan's bedside. Evan looked so peaceful, the most rested I'd ever seen him in quite some time. The weeks prior he was running around to doctors' appointments, taking calls from employees, and attempting to run his business, while all during this time, he had been extremely sick. As Dr. Sastoraki examined Evan I mentioned that Evan was moving his feet during the night, Dr. Sastoraki responded that it's not uncommon for the body to have movement, even when the individual is in an induced coma. Dr. Sastoraki, gently pulled Evan's eyelid up and shined a light, he moved to the other eye and did the same thing, shifting the light back and forth, closing the lid and once again, shining the light in the eye.

"Mrs. Mills, I'm going to schedule Evan for an MRI this morning, I'm not seeing any pupil reaction in Evan's eyes when I shine the light. His pupils should become smaller and larger depending on how much light is directed at the pupils, I'm concerned that he may have brain trauma." "Dr. Sastoraki, what do you mean brain trauma, how is this possible if he had the flu, bacteria, whatever we were dealing with?" "Mrs. Mills, we will know more once we have completed the test on Evan. At this time these are my suspicions, and I'd like to get Evans test completed as soon as possible." As Dr. Sastoraki left the room, I stood there dumfounded, "At what point did everything turn, how can Evan have brain trauma from this?" I walked over to Evan's bedside, and with all my will I pleaded with him to open his eyes, move his feet, do something to show me that he would be okay! I gently pushed his hair back from his forehead, please Evan, tell me where you are, I know that you're somewhere inside that body, please come out and show us the man that we all know and love.

A short time later, two hospital staff arrived to take Evan down for his test. The young tech looked at me "the test should run about a half hour, once all testing is complete, we will bring him back to his room and let you know." I walked back out to the waiting room. I knew I had to call Hailey; she was just as anxious about knowing what was going on with her dad as anyone. I played out in my mind, what and how I would tell her, I did not want to alarm her. "Hailey, good morning. They're running a few more tests on daddy this morning, he just went down for an MRI, just checking on his brain activity." I could not bring myself to tell her that the doctor said he may have brain trauma. It was taking all that I had to hold back the tears. I was so worried about Evan, worried about the kids. Not knowing exactly what I should tell them about their dads' condition. I did not want them to feel any of this pain. I wanted to shield them and help them in any way that I could.

I sat in the waiting room, recalling so much of my life together with Evan. We always seemed like the perfect match; he always balanced me out. He had a knack for putting things into perspective. The building could be burning down around him, and he would have that calm, take-charge attitude. All would get taken care of in due time, he would say, "Don't worry, Mallory, all will be fine." The only time I've seen Evan lose his cool is if it involved his family. It was always family first and foremost, which was a crazy balancing act with the business.

Evan always took care of his employees. If they needed something, he made sure they got it, one way or another. A few weeks before Christmas they were all given a nice bonus. If someone needed money before payday, Evan would cut them a check to help them out. Evan knew the struggles; he never wanted his employees to have to experience it if he could help it. The one thing Evan wanted was for his employees to always be upfront with him, no lying, and no stealing. That would have broken the trust between them.

I remember a time; it was in late November and Evan had found out that an employee had stolen fuel from the office. He drove out to his house, adamant that he was going to fire the guy on the spot. Evan couldn't understand why the guy just didn't come into his office and ask; the stealing part just didn't set well. As Evan knocked on the door a blonde-haired little boy about 6 years old answered the door. He looked at Evan and said, "look, I lost a tooth" with a wide grin you could see he was missing some of his baby teeth. All the anger and rage Evan felt towards that employee evaporated. Evan looked at the little boy "sorry buddy, I have the wrong house", and walked back to his truck to leave. Evan was a ball of emotions. He thought of this guy trying to be a good dad, keeping the home warm for his kids. It became a moment in Evan's life he wouldn't forget. He knew in his own life how hard his dad had to work to take care of their big family. This would be a situation that he would let go.

"Mrs. Mills, Evan is back in his room. The Neurologist would like to talk with you prior to going in to see him." As I walked back down the long hallway, I was praying it was going to be good news. I was directed into a small room to meet with the Neurologist. As I approached the desk, I could see an image on the screen. I knew this was related to Evan, the cloudy gray, white, and black clouds on the screen didn't make any sense to me. "Hi, Mrs. Mills, I'm Dr. Brijone. I've been reviewing Evan's MRI results, I'm very sorry, but it does not look good." There was no sugarcoating anything, Dr. Brijone was not pulling any punches. I could tell by his approach he was going to tell me like it was. As Dr. Brijone pointed at the various portions of the image, he explained what was going on with Evan's brain.

"Mrs. Mills, what Evan has is difficult to diagnose in its early stages, it could easily be identified as the flu without early detection with blood work. You had mentioned when Evan was admitted to the ER that he was diagnosed weeks prior by his providers' office as having the flu. His symptoms were fever, body aches, back pain, and little appetite." "In reviewing Evan's labs and the MRI results we have determined that he has a spinal infection." I'm looking at Dr. Brijone, with a confused look, "Dr. Brijone, if it's an infection why can't it just be treated with antibiotics?" "Mrs. Mills, this is a bacterial infection, called Staphylococcus aureus. If this had been caught and treated earlier, Evan may have had a fighting chance., At this time, Evan's brain is severely swollen. We can take him in for a procedure to reduce the pressure on his brain. The procedure would involve drilling at the top of Evan's head to release some of the fluid. I want you to know there are risks involved with this procedure, I can't say this will improve Evan's condition. I want you to take some time to think about this and discuss it with close family members. I'm sorry Mrs. Mills, I wish I had better news to deliver."

What did Dr. Brijone just say, they want to drill into the top of Evans skull and release the pressure from his brain? I walked into this hospital days ago, thinking, "this is it; Evan will now have a fighting chance. He is now at a hospital with highly skilled doctors and nurses, and they're going to save him." I had no idea what to make of this conversation I just had, none of it made sense to me.

I walked back to Evan's room; I slid the glass doors to the side and entered. I could see that someone had been in his room, a tiny Christmas tree had been placed near the window. My God, how this man loved Christmas. It was one of Evan's favorite holidays. I thought to myself, I hope I'm in the room when he opens his eyes and sees this, he is going to love it! He will be smiling from ear to ear. The condition the neurologist just presented to me was out the window. In my mind Evan was going to awaken to this amazing Christmas tree at his bedside. In my momentarily mental state of denial, I felt happy!

I sat next to Evan's bedside and took his hand. He looked tired today, his color was off, he had been fighting this infection for so long, and the results were not getting any better. I felt so selfish for telling him to keep on fighting, and telling him he was going to get better, telling him that the kids and I could not live without him. I could not imagine the unbearable pain he was in, his spine, his brain, the thought of drilling the top of his head sickened me. "Evan, help me, I want to make the best decisions for you, but I'm so afraid of losing you. Please just squeeze my hand. Let me know you hear me." As I watched Evan, I quietly prayed that I would see some movement from him.

I laid my head down on Evan's arm, envisioning how life had been, his strong arms hugging me. Not a time in our life did we pass each other without touching our hands together. The times I'd be in the kitchen cooking, music softly playing, and he would come in from work and just take me in his arms and slow dance. The arms I see today are thin, and frail, the numerous I.V. s hooked up, pumping every bit of fluid they could get into him to heal his body. I would move mountains to have you back just one more time, to let you know how grateful I am for all you did in my life and our children's. Evan please, open your eyes!

THE FAMILY ROCKED

Dr. Brijone wanted to meet with immediate family members at 10:00 a.m. the following morning, to discuss the plan for Evan. We were all under the impression that we were going to discuss the horrific drilling procedure to Evan's skull to release the pressure, and what we were to expect afterwards. Dr. Brijone walked into the conference room, he sat quietly for a moment before he began to talk. "We evaluated Evan throughout the night and had another MRI completed on his brain, there is very little brain activity, he is brain-dead. Evan has a 1% chance of survival. His organs are slowly failing, and the Staphylococcus aureus has invaded his body. Later today, we will be removing the mechanical ventilator. If he survives, we will be moving him to a nursing facility to provide him with long-term care." The room was so quiet, I don't think anyone was even breathing at this moment. We were just staring at one another in total disbelief with our mouths wide open.

I knew in my heart that there was no way in hell Evan would ever be okay with living his final days in a nursing home. I still could not believe we were even having this conversation, this could not be happening to Evan. I slowly stood up and looked at the family members gathered around the table. "I want everyone to respect my decisions in regard to Evan's care, this is very difficult, we all know that Evan would never want his life to be this way." As I looked around the table, I could see the tears and the slow nodding of heads in agreement. I don't know where I got the strength and courage to stand, but I felt if anything, I had to be Evan's voice going further.

This man that led such a private life, a humble caring man, this man that tied every string on his nursing gown before his physical, a man that would quickly wrap a towel around himself before I entered the bathroom. I could not see anyone caring for Evan besides me, he would be absolutely mortified with a stranger bathing or feeding him, it would never happen in my lifetime.

I sat in the waiting room as family members went in to visit Evan, we were all so devastated by the news. I looked down and put my head in my hands to avoid seeing the sadness on their faces. I picked up my phone and called my sister Payton, trying to hold back the tears as I told her, "Evan has only a 1% chance at survival.", I could hear Payton on the other end, a deep breath, and with complete sadness "I'm so sorry, Mallory." I felt completely broken. I don't think there was anything that anyone could say or do at that point; that would bring me out of this dark pit.

I continued to watch the door to the ICU as family members and close employees walked out sobbing. I hurt so badly for them, I wanted to say something, but I also wanted to be left alone. I was angry, angry that the hospital couldn't save Evan. Angry that Evan had to work so hard all his life and die so young. Evan did not deserve this. There were so many other losers in this world that I felt should die before Evan! "God, can't you see what a good man Evan is, let him stay, take someone else that is not grateful to be alive!"

I watched as one of Evan's employees walked out from the ICU, clearly shaken, tears streaming down his face. The same employee that called Evan over a week ago screaming his fucking head off! I could hear you screaming at Evan, I was sitting across the room and heard every bit of that conversation. You were apparently pissed about something again. I heard Evan repeatedly saying, "calm down" and then telling you to "go ahead and quit." This was a weekly occurrence with you. It wasn't the first time Evan dealt with this kind of shit from you, but certainly it would be his last! He will now be in peace, and no longer dealing with your childish meltdowns!" I was so angry at you; you could have made Evan's life easier! I wanted a bullhorn to blast out "I fucking hate you!"

As angry as I was at you, I couldn't stay mad at you. I know that Evan was like a father to you, he made a huge impact on your life. I know you respected him and appreciated all the opportunities in life that he helped you achieve. You were just young and immature, still finding your way in the world. You like me, would have to deal with losing someone that you loved. I knew you would have days where the heaviness in your heart felt like it was too much to bear. You will say a thousand times over, "I wish I had one more chance to talk to you."

I wanted to go back to Evan's room, but I also wanted to give Evan's family some privacy to sit with him and talk while he was still with us. The ICU door swung open, it was Susan, I started to head in thinking all the family members had left Evan's room. As I got near Evan's room I heard a voice, a crying, howling begging, pleading voice, it was Evan's younger brother Josh. Josh was hugging Evan, crying "Evan please, please don't die, I don't know what I'll do without you, please Evan, please." My knees buckled outside of Evan's room, my body slowly slid down the wall, and I just sat on the floor bawling my eyes out. There was nothing I could do to stop what was happening to Evan, all the hurt and pain the family was feeling was emotionally unbearable. I thought of Evan's mom, she was now in her late 80's, to outlive your child is not something a parent ever wants to endure in life. I thought of Evan's dad, whom Evan missed dearly after he passed, I know he would welcome Evan into Heaven with open arms.

God, please give our family strength to make it through this. Please guide Evan through Heavens gates into the arms of his dad to take him home!

A MOMENT TO REMEMBER

At Evan's bedside I sat with Hailey and Noah, listening to the rhythmic sound of all the mechanical equipment hooked up to him. I closed my eyes and rested my head on his chest. I knew they would be removing the ventilator soon, I just wanted to listen to Evan's heartbeat as long as I could. I wanted to remember this moment and the sound of his beating heart forever! If I closed my eyes and blocked out the other sounds it felt as if it was any other night for us, lying in bed, with my head on his chest. I liked this feeling, and I didn't want it to end, it was the closest I had felt to Evan in weeks. I reached for Evan's hand, he had lost so much weight, his strong hands felt so weak and frail in my hand. I rubbed his arm, hoping in some way this was comforting to him, hoping he knew we were there with him. Holding Evan's hand and listening to his heartbeat, I could have fallen asleep. It felt like it was normal, like at any second Evan would sit up and ask us, what was going on, and why was he here in the hospital.

I looked down at Hailey. She was massaging Evan's feet and ankles, his organs were slowly failing, his feet and ankles had swollen to twice their size. I could only imagine the heartache she was feeling at this moment knowing that her dad would soon be gone. I prayed that a miracle would occur when they removed the ventilator, and Evan would begin to breathe on his own. I looked at Noah, knowing he felt helpless, trying to be supportive of us in every way possible. Noah had been a trooper, right by our side the entire time, staying at the hospital one night so that I could go home to be with Bryan. I know Evan was accepting of Noah and thought of him as a son, we were both happy that eventually he would be marrying Hailey.

Our brief time of solitude with Evan was interrupted as Dr. Brijone slid the glass doors open. "Mallory, in a moment we will be removing the ventilator, we will give you some time with Evan but once we begin the process, we will have to ask you to leave the room." I nodded as though I understood, I just wasn't prepared, what if Evan quickly passed when the ventilator was removed? Before leaving the room, I had to ask Dr. Brijone, "is there a possibility that Evan will survive the night, how much longer do we have with him?" "Mallory, it's very difficult to say, it may be minutes, or hours, Evan has put up a good fight, but his organs are failing." I felt selfish, I wanted Dr. Brijone to wait, to delay the inevitable. I didn't know if Evan was in pain, and I didn't know the toll this had taken on his body. I just knew I did not want to see that heart beep on that screen to end!

  We gathered ourselves and left the room and proceeded to the ICU waiting room. We each looked at each other. I knew at that very moment each of us was doing all we could to hold it together. My eyes for a moment are fixated on Hailey, still wearing her scrubs from class, her eyes puffy, the bags under her eyes show that she had not slept in days, holding onto this vigil for her dad. We sat there in the ICU waiting area, just like so many other families had before us. We all prayed that Evan would still be with us once we returned to his room.

  It seemed like forever, when a young nurse came into the waiting area to let us know that we could return to Evan's room. I think we were all at a fast sprint to return to his room. I did not want to waste a moment of time; I did not want to be a second late to be back with Evan. As we walked into his room, strangely it was nice to see his face, it was no longer being strangled by the ventilator. I touched Evan's face and traced the deep lines left by the ventilator straps; I brushed his hair behind his ears. I noticed the stubble on Evan's face, this was a rarity, he was always clean shaving, just like his dad he shaved daily, like clockwork. I looked at the monitors, the slow rhythmic sound of his heartbeat was functioning on its own, I thanked God and prayed it would stay that way.

  I knew I had to eventually come to terms, knowing that if Evan made it through the night, he would be transported to a nursing home to be cared for, he was in a vegetive state and would require 24/7 care. It made me sick to my stomach to even think that this big strong man that stood 6'3", would now require daily nursing assistance from others. Evan was always the man that others came to for help. To envision this once capable man of now having to be hand fed and changed daily broke my heart. If this were to happen, it would be temporary, I would do everything in my power to make our home adaptable for Evans care.

It was as if Evan knew what the final outcome would be if he were to survive. As the evening progressed his vital signs continued to deteriorate. The rhythmic sound of his heart was now interrupted by slow, struggled breathing, his color turned to an ashy gray, and his ankles and feet, continued to swell. The ICU floor nurse popped in periodically, her last stop was two hours after Evan was removed from the ventilator and she advised us, "I'll call the hospital chaplain." We knew and she knew that Evan had very little time left.

As the hospital chaplain administered Evan's last rights, I knew Evan was no longer in pain. I prayed that his reunion in heaven was a glorious one. That his dad was standing there smiling and giving him the biggest hug, happy that once again he was with his boy. I prayed that his two other brothers that were deceased prior would be standing in a huddle, all together, talking about football, baseball and all their other favorite sports. These were the only thoughts in my head that would allow me to think it was okay that Evan left us. That he would be joined by others that loved him as much as us. I did not want to have any bad thoughts of the prior week. I now wanted Evan to have peace, to feel the love of the ones he had lost so many years ago.

I grabbed the Christmas tree and white hospital bag that contained Evan's things. I thought of the day he went to the hospital; he was so worried about what he was wearing. For the life of me I couldn't understand why he would even care. Did he know in some way that this was how his hospital visit would end? It was hard for me to wrap my head around it. I knew exactly what was in that white plastic bag, his favorite outfit.! The clothes that he put on every day, no matter if he was meeting the president of a bank or the CEO of a company. Evan was not the "dress to impress" type. He didn't have to be. Evan was a brilliant man with skills and knowledge in his field which could not be matched by a college graduate. As my grandfather always said, "Clothes don't make the man!"

I walked out to my car in the parking garage. What had it been, 2, 3 days ago, that I had parked here? I had lost all track of time. For me it seemed like I had been at that hospital for months. I opened the passenger side door and set the Christmas tree down on the seat along with the white hospital bag. As soon as I got in the car, I pulled everything out of the white bag. I smiled as I looked at the dark blue t-shirt and Dickies. The man that wore the same clothes to a luxury car dealership to surprise me with a new car for my birthday, only to be ignored by the salesmen.

I remember him calling me, "Mallory, I want to buy you this car, but none of the salesmen will give me the time of day here." I could only laugh because my Evan, the business owner that would put on his dark blue T-shirt and Dickies every day showed up with me at the dealership later that day. I didn't think we were going in there tonight to buy a car. I thought Evan was going to string them along and walk out the door. A young salesman approached us. I see Evan smiling and shaking his hand. This young salesman was a former employee of Evans. He had recently left our company to go back to college full-time during the day. He told Evan he was working there part-time a few nights a week to help cover college costs.

Evan found his salesman! Evan looked at him and said, "Perfect, we're here to buy a car tonight. Mallory, show him the car that you want." It was four steps later and I was standing next to the show room model! As we walked out the door with our sales receipt, the other salesmen were looking at us. Evan looked at them, waived the sales receipts in the air and said, "and that's how it's done!"

I turned on the ignition. The radio was still streaming Christmas music. I had been listening to the same radio station ever since this whole nightmare with Evan began. The music was so calming. It always brought me back to some of the best times at Christmas. I looked over at the passenger seat with the small, decorated Christmas tree. I really thought that eventually Evan would have woken up and seen that tree by his bedside. I knew that as soon as the spring brought warmer weather, I'd plant it in our yard in memory of Evan.

Come to me, all you who are weary and burdened, and I will give you rest.

Matthew 11:28

WILL THAT BE A LA CARTE?

I know I had depended on Evan's sister Sarah so much after Evan had passed. If it hadn't been for her, I really don't know where I would have ended up. This was her brother, and I know deep down inside she felt she needed to be here for me, it's what Evan would have wanted. To go through the trauma of all the events at the hospital together, I felt she had a strong understanding of where I was mentally and emotionally. We didn't have to talk. Just a quick text from her every day to check on the family was reassuring. I know there were days I just wanted to cover my head and stay in bed. The only thing that kept me going was my kids. Sarah would be my driving force to push me each day to make decisions that I did not want to make or to acknowledge at all, the ones that needed to be made.

As Sarah and I pulled into the cemetery, I looked around at the perfectly placed gray headstones, it was late April, and if not for the spring flowers popping up from the ground, this place would have felt so cold and unwelcoming. This cemetery held the remains of so many of Evan's family members. I would have loved to have Evan right near his parents, but they had purchased their plot years ago, and at this time, real estate near them was non-existent. In my heart, I knew that Evan needed a quiet peaceful place to be laid to rest. He had worked hard his entire life, long hours, and weekends, taking care of so many people. It was his time for peace and quiet, no phone ringing, no employees complaining or customer calling, and no longer playing the family peacekeeper.

I wanted to do my best to find a burial plot for Evan. I continued to gaze over the small area's that had a plot open. I had been looking for hours, I finally found a spot where there were no other headstones around. The plot was secluded and quiet, at the base of the cemetery hill, with thick green grass, and lots of bright sunshine. There would never be trees blocking the warm sun that would fall on his gravestone daily. I knew Evan would have wanted this spot.

The warm sun and silence took me back to his family's large kitchen, it was surrounded by windows that allowed the sun to flow in all day. The family kitchen where Evan would sit for hours with his dad and brothers talking and planning out their day together. This room was always comforting to me, the warmth and love I felt were immediate when I walked into that room. This place for Evan would hold all that love and warmth, just like it had in his childhood home.

Sarah and I walk over to the caretaker, I was familiar with Toby and had often seen him around in our community. Toby had lived here his entire life and knew Evan's family very well; he had attended school with Evans younger brother Josh. Toby approached Sarah and I, he began to tell me that I picked out one of the best spots in the cemetery. He looked at us and smiled, "The rainfall drains down the hill, and the bright summer sun keeps that grass nice and green, "it's the perfect spot you would want to come and visit, to sit in the sun and rest your feet in the grass."

As we walked with Toby, he looked at me and said apologetically, "Mallory, if you want that plot for Evan, we will need a deposit from you today. I turned to him and said, "Toby, there is not a chance in hell I would let this plot go. I'll be paying you in full!" As Toby followed me to the car, I wrote out the check for $450.00. From this day forward this will be Evan's little piece of heaven.

I walked with Toby back to Evan's plot. I watched as Toby carefully placed a metal stake with a blue-ribbon marking Evans plot. Toby began to explain to me that within the next few months, I would get the deed for Evan's plot, and keep it in a secure place for our family records. I did not want to hear Toby saying all of this. We were too young to be here doing this! "Thank you, Toby. I came here today for one thing, a beautiful, peaceful resting spot for Evan."

I pulled my jacket tightly around me and quickly walked towards Sarah's car. The weather had changed drastically within the last hour. The rain and wind made it difficult to stay warm. It was only a week ago I was driving with the windows down with temps in the high 70s, mother nature just couldn't make up her mind. I slid into the passenger seat and breathed a sigh of relief; thinking I just made it over the first difficult hurdle of many. I kept thinking if I just held my breath, jumped over all these hurdles, and continued to act like things were normal to me, none of it would be real. I knew that once I endured the torture today, I would go home to see Evan.

Sarah, looked over at me, gave me a nod, and acknowledged that Evan will love the spot I had picked out for him. I just nod in agreement, not wanting to talk, this had been difficult for both of us. As Sarah continued to look at me, I could tell that whatever it was she wanted to say was killing her to say it. "Do you think you're ready for our appointment at the funeral home?" It was though I was getting my que from a movie director, there were no feelings or emotions to my response. "Yes, I am." I'm in autopilot, I was going to remain emotionless. If I open myself up, I may not be able to go to the funeral home. I just know I need to get this done; I want to go home. At home I can go in my room, I can cry, I can set aside this false façade, that all is okay in my world.

We drove in silence to the funeral home, the only sound was the swishing of the wiper blades on the windshield, damn rain. I hated the cold weather. I remember always asking Evan why he wouldn't open a branch in a warmer climate, his response always was, "Mallory, that would be another headache that would take me hundreds of miles away from my family! I have enough on my plate here." So here we would live for eternity in Upstate NY, enduring every freezing cold winter.

We finally arrive at the funeral home and pull into the parking lot, dejavu hits me. I tell myself I have been here a thousand times. Its different today, today I am the client. I'm the one that is planning the funeral for a loved one, this is the last place I want to be. I know it's going to take a lot to get through this appointment, because again, it's one more thing to remind me that Evan is gone. My mind will continue to fight me on this and throw memories up all during the meeting. The memories and discussions of Evan create the most pain, the more it is thrown in my face the more I attempt to deny it. I freeze up with fear, to realize I am once again on my own.

The funeral home is in Evan's hometown, it is a quaint small town, tree's line the streets, mom and pop restaurants, and a handful of coffee shops here and there. Evan attended the high school just down the road from the funeral home. Evan and I had been here so many times throughout the years for family and friends' services. The interior of the funeral home is old and dated. The beige wallpaper with faded, small blue flowers is slightly lifting at the edges. The soft brown suede chairs fit snugly in the corners of each wall. As I walked down the long dark-paneled hallway, the smell of old musty carpet with a hint of vanilla filled my nose. This place brought back so many sad memories of people that had passed way too young or finally joined their long-lost mate at a decrepit age.

As Sarah and I made our way down the long hallway, we are directed into an office by an older gentleman. The gentleman introduces himself as Mr. Stilner, a tall older man, with thick glasses, dark hair slicked back with a ting of gray around his face, He comes across as though he may have been doing this his entire life. He proceeds to sit down and motions for Sarah and me to sit down across from him.

Mr. Stilner hands me a thick folder with a beautiful image of the funeral home on the front cover. Within the folder I would find every detail of what to expect, and what the funeral home would need from me. I pulled out the packet of paperwork and listened as Mr. Stilner did his talk. As he went on about all the various options that were available for Evan's funeral. I felt sick to my stomach everything about planning a funeral was like ordering off a menu, do I want the Filet Mignon or the Cheeseburger with fries' option for Evans funeral?

As Mr. Stilner went on with the Ala'carte cost, my mind began to drift off, I looked at the walls and the old over-stuffed furniture. How many families prior to me sat in this same chair making the same decisions that I was making? How many of these people were thinking, "how will I pay for the funeral cost?" Would they have to max out a credit card, dip into their savings or sell-off whatever they could to come up with the money! My heart broke thinking of these families and having to make these types of decisions at such a painful and vulnerable time.

    I could hear the continued drippling of Mr. Stilners voice, Oak Casket, Memorial Cards, Memorial Candle, a non-stop looping video of Evan's life, guest book, blah, blah, blah. I think I lost track of the cost at $8,000.00; I know Evan would never want the Filet Mignon menu option but, dammit he was going to get it, he deserved it! This man was a saint to me, he saved me in so many ways there would be no way for me to ever show him my gratitude then this! If I had the energy and could deal with people I'd throw him a fucking parade, he deserved it!

    Mr. Stilner slides the contract over to me. I think at that moment my eyes and mouth may have given away my shock and surprise, "$10,000?" Mr. Stilner is quick to explain to me that they can cut some costs. In my head, I'm saying "No, no, no, I'm keeping the Filet Mignon menu option!" "Mrs. Mills, there is also a payment plan option, this is something you may want to consider, if the cost is something that you are not able to come up with at this time." In my head the voices were screaming, "Wow, Mr. Stilner, you are giving me every possible reason to go with the Filet Mignon menu option, slightly telling me you will accommodate me in any way possible to pile on all the AlaCarte extras!" Thankfully, Evan had a small Life Insurance Policy that would make it possible for me to lighten the financial hardship, so I was sticking with Filet Mignon! I replied, "Mr. Stilner, I am fine. I can cover the cost!"

    I could not shake that sick feeling in my gut. How can this make any sense at all? It's not enough that families are grieving over the loss of their loved one, but on top of that they are put in a position of financial hardship. Who in the hells wants that monthly reminder as they write a check that they lost their loved one! It gives the brain the opportunity to ramp up every month, it gets those memories and emotions in high gear. The anxiety and fear come flooding back in again like a tidal wave crashing, now you're in a full-blown panic attack.

As sickening as it was with all the exuberant cost and AlaCarte options, I'm sure families had no other choice but to go with the Cheeseburger and Fries, when in their heart they knew full well their loved one deserved the Filet Mignon and so much more. I believe when we lose someone, we always think we could have done so much more when they were alive. That same guilt makes us go overboard, overindulging for their funeral thinking we are showing them so much love.

That is exactly how I felt when planning Evans funeral, I went overboard because of the guilt. In my head I felt spending all this money on his funeral was my way of saying how much I truly loved and respected him for all that he did for our family. How hard he worked but never let on to others the stress he was going through. The many times he cut a vacation short to go back to the office to work. The weekends he missed with the guys golfing because he was at the office coordinating jobs for the following week. The hours of sleep he missed dealing with running a company that operated 24/7. I could go on forever, and if that folder mentioned anything about erecting a monument in a loved one's name, dammit Evan would have one! I don't care I would sell the friggen farm to honor this man.

As I'm walking out of the funeral home, I'm feeling pissed, sad, and every emotion you can name. I wondered, how could anyone do this job, walking in this door every single day. To me this would be heart-wrenching. To just stand silently by and watch the family members gather around their deceased loved one, to meet with them to discuss all the AlaCarte costs, to tell them that burying their family member is going to cost thousands of dollars. To tell the family members repeatedly "I'm sorry, I'm really sorry, here's a tissue." I guess I just don't understand the funeral business. It was time for me to get the hell out of here!

Mr. Stilner catches me at the end of the hallway, "Mrs. Mills, I know this is not easy, but we will need a photo of Evan, and the obituary write-up by Monday morning, you can email it to us. Once we receive those things, we will work with the newspaper to get his obituary published. Also, on Monday please drop off the clothing you would like Evan to be laid to rest in, you may also include personal items in his coffin." As Mr. Stilner rambled on my mind drifted off and could only focus on what Evan would want in his coffin. He is not a child, maybe pictures of his children, maybe some of the pictures of him with his dad at the horse track, my god, do I even have a recent photo of Evan, he hated his picture taken! The clothes, hell if it were up to Evan, it would be a T-shirt and Dickies.

I slammed the funeral home door behind me as I left. I felt I had come here, done what needed to be done. No more talking about it!

That evening after Bryan went to bed I started working on Evan's obituary. To put Evan's accomplishments in life in one paragraph was not going to work. I poured my heart out in Evan's obituary, the world needed to know what a wonderful man they had lost. The best father and one of the most gracious bosses/employers you would ever want to meet. I finished off what I felt was the sincerest form of gratitude to Evan, a loving obituary. I hit the send button, and off it went to Mr. Stilner.

The following morning, I got up before the sound of the alarm. As I walked down the hallway, I recall always smelling the coffee brewing before we got out of bed. I missed that smell. I had stopped making a large pot of coffee since Evan had passed. I was dumping most of the pot out each day, now I used a single serve cup. I set my cup down, pushed start, I waited for the coffee to whirl into my cup. The lingering smell of the coffee brewing was like magic to my nostrils. How I wished Evan was here with me to have a cup of coffee. I knew that today was going to be a rough day. Today was the day that I would pick out Evan's headstone. I wanted to do this alone!

I got Bryan up and made him some breakfast, French toast sticks, and strawberry yogurt, he was a creature of habit, he did not like change. "You're going over to Colby's house today, while I run some errands, so get yourself going." I never told Bryan where I was going or what I was working on for Evan's funeral, I wanted to protect him and act like everything was okay. I thought I was presenting the strongest front for him, like if I didn't acknowledge it, then it never happened.

I pulled up to Lexie's house to drop off Bryan. Lexie came over to my car to talk. "Are you going to be okay today?" Me in my best voice of denial said, "of course!" "If you need someone to go with you, you know that I'll go." "Lexie, I'll be fine, thank you for watching Bryan." Again, having a conversation about what I was doing, made me more aware that I had to acknowledge that Evan was not here. The more it was pressed the more I became upset. I rolled up my car window and knew this conversation just couldn't continue, I'd be a blatting idiot with Bryan standing nearby, the alarms in his 10-year-old brain would be going off.

As I drove, I had my normal conversation with Evan in the car, always trying to figure out, if what I was doing was the best for me and the kids. Always just asking him to give me the strength to get through this, to help me be brave for our kids. I was always looking for some form of confirmation that it all would be okay and that he approved of what I had done so far. As I pulled in the parking lot, I told Evan that I was picking him out the best stone in the place that memorialized his life in every way.

The company I had chosen for Evan's headstone was located on a busy stretch in a local city. I had passed this business several times and always admired how beautiful the stones looked, always shiny, the granite and marble were remarkable. I knew this would be the place where I would be getting Evans headstone. There was one particular headstone that stood out in the front lawn of the business. It was a black, shiny headstone with white letters and graphics etched into it. This headstone stood out from all the gray stones in the yard, it made me think of the first day I pulled into the cemetery to pick out Evans plot. All the gray headstones popped up everywhere, there was a little color from the spring flowers, it just seemed so drab and depressing at the cemetery. This black headstone would be exactly what Evan would have wanted.

I was running my fingers over the smooth granite and admiring how pretty the stone was when I was suddenly startled by a voice behind me "I see you are admiring the Indian Black Granite headstone, it's a beautiful stone isn't it?" "Yes, it is, I'm looking for a headstone for my husband." "It's one of our best sellers here. It has a beautiful sleek look to it. Would you like to come in the office, we can see if this is the one for you?" I replied, "Sure, and this is the ONE for me."

As I entered the office, I see piles of small samples of stone here and there on the other office desk. The pictures on the walls show how magnificent these stones are, they are so beautifully adorned by flowers across the top. They had different styles fonts, and pictures. It appeared you could get pretty detailed with your selection. I knew with Evan that it would be simple, but it would represent something he loved.

"So, you're set on the Indian Black stone?" I knew even before I got there that my mind was set on the Indian Black stone, I didn't need to look at any other options. "Yes, I'm set on the Indian black stone!" As we sat down and discussed all the options, I once again felt that, yes there are choices, but for every choice and option, it will cost you more money. At this point I knew the entire process; I just must accept it; funerals are expensive and there is no way around it. Unless of course, I did what Evan mentioned to me so many times in the past. "Mallory, just dig a hole outback and bury me, I don't give a shit what happens to me after I'm dead!" He certainly was a character!

"Do you have any ideas on graphics for the stone? We will do a laser cut; it will come out very precise and clean." I had thought about the headstone the prior evening, I had dreamt about it also. Evan and I were back at the beach just staring out watching the waves roll in, the salty ocean air blowing Evan's hair in the wind. We stood there for the longest time, holding hands, and just enjoying the spectacular view, mentioning to one another how peaceful it was. I knew this would be the graphic I wanted on the headstone. Now all I needed to do is communicate this clearly so that we were all happy in the end.

"Mrs. Mills, you have picked out a beautiful stone. The process will take about 6 weeks to complete, we will make arrangements to set it at your husband's grave soon after that." I did not like the thought of Evan not having his headstone when he was laid to rest, but I was asking for a custom stone, and ultimately, Evan would love it. All I needed to do now was put 50% down so that they could start the process. I handed him a check for $3,500.00 and headed out the door. It had been a long afternoon; I just wanted to close my eyes and go back to the evening before and replay my dream in my head, that beautiful beach with Evan by my side.

On my way home, I received a call from Mr. Stilner from the funeral home. He received the email and said the obituary was wonderful." Mallory, due to the length it will cost $700.00 to run it in its entirety." "Mr. Stilner, Evan is worth every penny of that, run it in its entirety!" "Also, Mrs. Mills, just a reminder, can you please drop off Evans rest attire this evening or early tomorrow morning so that we are fully prepared for his service?" "Absolutely!"

Throughout this entire week I had noticed my emotions and responses were very robotic. I was systematically going through a checklist in my mind. I was not going to let any outside distractions stop me from doing what needed to be done. I was not going to let any emotional breakdowns get in my way, I know Evan would have wanted me to be strong and push through this process. I was giving my family and friends very little of my time, not allowing them to ask me too many questions. I had closed and tightened the hatch on my emotions, and I was hoping I could keep it that way.

I pulled into Lexie's driveway, she was outside with the boys and came over to my car. "Lexie, would you mind if Bryan stays for dinner, I have to bring Evan's rest attire to the funeral home and I really don't want Bryan to go with me?" "Of course, take your time and get done what you need to do, he can stay with us." I was just so thankful for Lexie's friendship; she was there for me and had helped me so much with Bryan. I think Lexie knew I did not want to sit down and talk with her about Evan or anything that had been going on the past few days.. Once everything calms down and I'm in a better place I'll make it a point to get together.

    I went home and pulled out some of Evans old suits from our closet and decided on a gray suit with a light blue dress shirt. Evan always looked so handsome in that suit when he wore it. I thought back to Hailey planning her wedding and the opportunity to finally have a professional family photo of us together. We had some great photos, but not one of us as a family. Evan always seemed to duck out when it was picture time, but there was no avoiding it at Hailey's wedding.

    I folded the suit and set it to the side, I grabbed his black dress shoes and black socks, and as I was walking out of our bedroom, I remembered his wedding band. Evan had not worn his wedding band in years, he had broken his finger playing football several years ago, and the knuckle on his finger was never the same after that. He could no longer get it back on his finger after the injury healed.

    I arrived at the funeral home just before dusk, and Mr. Stilner met me at the door. I felt I had to explain to Mr. Stilner about Evans wedding band, he assured me that they would work with the local jeweler to fit it to Evans ring finger. I handed the bag of clothing to Mr. Stilner and just as it left my fingers I said, "Wait, I don't want you to put the socks or dress shoes on Evan, he hated getting dressed up, this is his day, and he would prefer it this way!" "Of course, Mrs. Mills we will do exactly that." As far back as I could remember, Evan was a man of comfort, not fashion, when he was at home, he would prefer sandals or go barefoot. I was done at the funeral home! I walked out to my car thinking, "is this really what Evan would have wanted, am I doing it for him or everyone else that is still living?"

    I called Lexie on my way home to let her know I'd be there soon to pick up Bryan. I felt so bad for Bryan, it was so late, we were all exhausted. I just wanted to pick him up, go home and forget this entire day. Bryan hopped in the car, talking non-stop about all that he and Colby had done that day. "Mom, do you think that Colby can come to our house tomorrow?" I didn't want to tell Bryan but tomorrow we would be going out to pick up his suit for the funeral. "Sure, he can come over for a little while tomorrow." I will deal with whatever comes my way tomorrow, but for now, I wanted Bryan to be a happy little boy, to laugh with his friend and not have to think about his father no longer being in our home when we get there.

I sent a quick text to Lexie, asking if Colby could come over tomorrow, even if it was for an hour. I did not for a second want to think what was ahead of Bryan the next few days, our families' emotions were all over the place. Hailey kept herself busy and really did not say too much. I believe we were all dealing with Evan's death the best that we could.

The following morning, Bryan woke up early, he knew that Colby was going to come to our house today. The boys played as Lexie, and I sat in the kitchen having a cup of coffee. It felt odd trying to carry on a conversation without bringing up Evan. Lexie knew it wasn't the best time, I think if the flood gates opened today, there would be no closing them. The only information I felt comfortable sharing was about the headstone, how beautiful it was and how it was perfect for Evan. I knew as soon as I mentioned it to Lexie, she would become emotional. I did not want Bryan to see anyone crying in our home, it triggered way too many emotions. "Okay, Lexie, Ive got to get Bryan moving, I have to find him a suit for tomorrow, thanks again for bringing Colby over for a little while, I'll talk to you later." I know I was cutting her visit short, but I did not want to chance any further discussion about Evan.

WHO MAKES PLANS?

Evan and I had been married for over 8 years before we even discussed having a Will. That conversation only came up because we were going on a cruise and our daughter Hailey would be staying back with my mom. Our attorney had mentioned it several times over the years, but we just somehow never had the time or honestly didn't think we needed a Will. We were both young, what could happen?

We finally planned to meet with our attorney one week prior to our scheduled cruise date. Of all the information that was gathered and put in our Will, the one area I struggled with was, who do you want to be your child's guardian should something happen to you? Our family combined was big, but they all have children of their own. Some were enjoying their freedom, and others just didn't seem like they could financially handle raising another child.

All our material possessions were easily distributed or determined to be sold off and put in a trust for Hailey but deciding on our most important possession. Our child was not going to be an easy decision. As a parent, you always feel there is no one in this world that can or will love your child as much as you do. I remember that day, looking over at Evan and saying, "We have to live until Hailey is at least 18 so that she can be independent and thrive on her own!" Evan looked at me and said, "Mallory, Will you stop? We are both young and healthy!"

We left our attorney's office that day without any guardian listed for Hailey. We felt we needed to think about this overnight and would let our attorney know the following morning. This was not going to be as easy as we thought it would be.

That evening at home, we asked Hailey, "who is your favorite person you love to spend time with?" Hailey, only thinking of the one person that would let her get away with murder and cover for her, blurted out, "Grandma." In our eyes, we were thinking of someone a little younger, someone that could stay up past 8:00 p.m., someone that had other hobbies besides hitting the Casino on the weekend.

As Evan and I lay in bed that evening, Evan said "Mallory, what about Penny and Stuart, they have no children and are financially secure, they would love Hailey as much as we do." I thought about it for a moment, "Evan, I think that arrangement would be the best for Hailey should anything happen to us." We had finally found what we felt was the perfect guardians for Hailey.

Evan's older brother Stuart and his wife Penny were never able to have children. Their home was in the same school district that Hailey attended, both had great jobs and a stable home life. We decided to reach out to Stuart and Penny in the morning to see if they would be willing to accept this huge responsibility!

After Hailey left for school we touched base with Stuart and Penny. We were not sure how they would respond, they never had children. Would they want to accept all the responsibility that came with raising a child? At this point in their lives maybe they had decided on having a quiet household. Maybe they had plans for an early retirement. All the scenarios started playing out in my head, what if they said no, who was our backup? I never realized how stressful this would be until faced with deciding who would be a huge part of my child's life if we should die.

It did not take Stuart and Penny that long to decide. They were ecstatic that we would have thought of them to be there for Hailey if anything should ever happen to us. I knew we had made the right choice; I could see how happy this made them. Stuart and Penny loved all their nieces and nephews and always made time to spend with them. They would get the nieces and nephews together to decorate Christmas cookies, throw a Halloween party, and have the occasional pizza and movie night. They loved having the kids over. At the end of the night, popcorn was everywhere, but they would sit there with smiles on their faces and say, "it was a great night."

It was a relief to have that huge weight lifted off my shoulders, and still, in my mind, I felt we would grow old gracefully watching Hailey raise children of her own. To me, this "Will" thing was just a formality!

Throughout the years, Evan and I had so many conversations about our own mortality. If I passed first or he was to pass first, what would the other do? I always wanted Evan to know he was to go on with his life. I could not see him staying home lonely, sad, and grieving for me for the rest of his life. I wanted him to remain happy. I wanted him to be emotionally stable and involved in his children's life. I could never see Evan turning to drugs or alcohol to soothe his sorrows, but I have seen it happen to families after trauma. I just hoped and prayed it would never happen to us.

Evan always joked that if I were to go first, he would have to hire backup to help him in the home with the kids and household chores. He always threw in "Mallory. I'm going first, so I'll never have to worry about any of that!" In a perfect world, the way I would want it to be, the two of us in our late 80's, laying in our bed, holding hands, going to sleep, and never waking up. I have read stories like this. It would be such a beautiful thing to live a long life together and leave the world at the same time. There would be no grieving, no loneliness, just pure bliss to be with the one you love forever, walking hand and hand through those pearly gates.

DENIAL

I remember the painful morning after Evan had passed. I had gotten home from the hospital a little after 2:00 a.m. and tried to fall asleep. I wanted to be up and dressed before Bryan woke up. I was not sure I would ever fall asleep at all. I had no idea how I was going to tell Bryan that his dad had passed away. In my head I ran a million scenarios repeatedly, trying to find the right words to keep this young man's heart from breaking.

I did not wake up the next morning until 8:00 a.m. I heard noises out in the dining room and wondered who was at our home so early. My mom had left when I got home from the hospital, so it had to be Bryan awake. I walked out to the dining room, and I see Bryan picking up all the loose paper from the dining room table. He had everything organized and picked up. He heard me coming down the hall and smiled, "Mom, look I finished it! What do you think of this Lego eating Whale?" He laughed and proceeded to tell me, "Eating the Lego people was dad's idea! I can't wait to show him!"

I looked at him with tears rolling down my face, "Bryan you did a fabulous job on that whale. Your dad would be so proud of you. Let's go in the living room, I want to talk to you about daddy." "Mom, why are you crying? Is dad, okay?"

I sat on the couch with Bryan, I looked at our family pictures on the walls. What I see on those walls today can never be recreated again. Any celebration in life that we may have missed will never present itself to us again. Those moments in life for us, are now gone. Our wedding picture, pictures with the kids, pictures of us at the beach, from here on out, Evan would no longer be captured in our life. It did not seem possible. He was always here for us.

I took a deep breath and prepared myself for whatever questions Bryan was going to ask me. He slides up on the couch next to me "Mom, how is dad feeling? Will he be coming home soon?" That was it, I couldn't hold back the tears, this boy for the past week had thought his dad was in the hospital dealing with the flu and would be home soon. As I tried to find the best way to tell Bryan I could feel my throat tighten. With a slight crack in my voice, I began, "Bryan, your dad was very, very sick. He did not get better at the hospital; he went to heaven with poppa last night." "Mom, what do you mean? Did dad die like that singer on television?"

    Bryan was correlating the death of Prince to what happened to his dad. The news of the singer's death was playing non-stop for the past two weeks, I hadn't even realized Bryan was watching it. I explained to Bryan the best way that I could, using words that I felt would give Bryan a better understanding, yet keeping in mind he was only ten-years old. I wanted him to know his dad was fighting hard to get better, but his body couldn't handle the illness.

    Bryan ran to his room, I could hear him crying from the living room, each sob was like a stab to my heart. I went to his room to see if I could console him. Bryan was under his blankets, his hands clutching the top edge of the blanket close to his body, his knees and legs curled up in a ball. As much as I tried to talk to Bryan, the more he shrank away from me, "mom, I want to be alone!" There was nothing in this world that I wanted more than to make things right for Bryan and take away his pain. As I walked down the hall, I could hear Bryan screaming over and over, "I hate this, I hate this!" I whispered back "I hate this also." This was too much traumatic information for a child to absorb.

    I sat back down on the couch, shaking my head, "there is no way in hell Evan is dead." We had made plans for our future together. "God, do you hear me, big plans dammit!" We have our annual family trip to Maine, there is absolutely no way Evan would ever want to miss our trip! His desk has got to be full of office work by now! Look, his cell phone is still ringing, and customers are calling to schedule jobs. Evan, you would never miss a call! "Evan, do you even realize all the sports you're missing? You could be sitting in your big comfy chair watching sports on your big screen television." We still have that big pot of homemade chicken noodle soup for you. I have so much to talk to you about, Hailey and Bryan, and all that's going on in their life right now. Dammit, Evan, there is no way on God's green earth that this could be happening, this is a nightmare, and when we all wake up, all will be back to normal!" I felt myself, attempting to wheel and deal, as though something would bring Evan back.

I sat on the couch and cursed everyone for making our lives turn out this way. I picked up the phone and called Evan's primary doctor. When Evan's doctor finally got on the phone I was screaming, "Do you know what it was like telling my 10-year-old son his father died! This was not the fucking flu!" I did not stop, I was angry, they could have done more! I took a breath, and I heard him respond, "Mallory, I am so sorry to hear about Evan. I wish we had done more or knew more at the time. This is an incredibly horrible situation for a child to deal with, I'm sorry." "Your apology will never make a difference, nor will it ever bring Evan back! I will have to deal with this along with my children for the rest of our lives! I can't sleep, I can't eat, my anxiety is so high right now I think my heart is beating out of my chest!" "Mallory, I think it would be best if we put you on something for a couple of months, I'm going to prescribe Valium."

I was so pissed hearing him tell me he was now going to put me on a drug I knew nothing about. A drug I felt he wanted to prescribe to me to numb my brain until I got over this "Did you just hear me say I have a 10-year-old son? How am I supposed to function like a normal parent on Valium!" I am now the ONLY parent, save your drugs!" I hung up the phone.

The days dragged on, and as difficult as it was, I was trying my best to get through everyday life! Every decision and event that occurred after Evan's death was like playing a part in a movie, and nothing seemed real. It was almost like watching a traumatic movie and wanting to rescue the victim. You could see and feel how tired, mentally, and emotionally drained they are, but you are helpless, there is nothing you can do to stop this movie, you are frozen with fear. You stand there emotionless, nodding your head, following the herd, hoping someone is leading you in the right direction. The problem is, "who is the leader? Are they also as fucked up as I am with the loss of Evan?" Are they strong enough leaders to get us through this and not breakdown?

Everything that was happening in our lives seemed to be happening at warp speed. I remember just staring at people at Evans funeral, not really hearing what they were saying. I could feel them hugging me, but I had no emotions or feelings. I was like a zombie, just standing there numb. I was thinking about Bryan, I had argued with him earlier, he was adamant that he was not going to his father's funeral. "Mom, I don't want to see dad like that, I'm not going. I want to remember him like he was before he went into the hospital." Sobbing he ran away to his room saying, "I don't want to see him dead." I did not force Bryan to go, I also did not want his last memory of his dad to be one that haunted him as a young child.

I would get phone calls and text messages, and I didn't know exactly how to respond to my family and friends. I let so many of them go unanswered. I didn't want company, I didn't want to have a conversation, and I certainly did not want to acknowledge in any way that Evan was gone. This denial would go on for months until it took its toll on me, physically and mentally. I knew in my mind that I had been in denial for so long, that it became second nature to think and feel that what I was doing, was somehow okay with Evan.

I remember in July, I had taken Bryan to Lego Land, it was to get away and celebrate his birthday. To me this was another milestone without Evan. I knew Evan was gone but I was still unwilling to accept it. This was our first trip that was a considerable distance from home. I made all the arrangements to ensure that we were picked up from the airport and delivered directly to the resort. I still had that fear of not having someone by my side to protect me and my son. I wanted to make sure that without Evan I was taking every precaution to keep Bryan and myself safe. I never had that fear when traveling with Evan. Now every bit of me was on high alert!

This trip is exactly what Bryan and I needed, he was completely entranced by the place. Everywhere you looked there was piles and piles of Legos to build with. My only hope for this trip was to see Bryan having fun and playing again like he always had with his dad. I figured tying in the Legos resort would provide Bryan with some great memories. I watched as Bryan built all kinds of crazy things, dance at the kid's parties at night, have breakfast with the characters and swim in a pool filled with Lego blocks. The laughs and smiles from Bryan reinforced my decision that this was a good trip for both of us.

As our last day approached, Bryan and I hung out by the pool, he had made some friends and was having a blast. I watched him laughing and splashing with the other kids, jumping off the foam Lego blocks, this was something I hadn't seen him do in months. I picked up my cellphone and took a picture of him laughing like crazy. I started typing a text message "Bryan is having such a great time, look at him" I pushed the send button and off it to went Evan.... The moment I realized what I had done I felt sick to my stomach. It was during that split second that I had forgotten that Evan was gone. All I wanted to do was show Evan that Bryan was finally laughing and smiling like a little boy again, he was not in his bedroom crying with the blankets pulled over his head.

This would not be the first time, nor the last time my mind would play a cruel joke on me. I had read so much on grief, and somewhere I had read that our brain is wired for connection, but trauma rewires them for protection. Everything I had been doing and feeling did not seem right at times. I was slipping up due to my brain trying to protect me from the trauma. I can see where denial was once again a way for me to protect myself and the kids from reality. In all honesty it was just prolonging me from dealing with Evans death head-on!

RIPPLE EFFECT

That evening I lay in bed, and the one thing I knew for certain was that I no longer wanted to deal with or be a part of the business that we had worked so hard to make successful!

Every ounce of my being blamed Evans death on that place. I strongly felt that Evan ran himself into the ground running that business, never allowing himself time to go to the doctor or take a sick day when he needed it. Every vacation we planned was interrupted and ended short! I cringe at the thought of Evan being at home, sick and the phone ringing non-stop or going to a doctor's appointment and the non-stop fucking ringing! The employees that called and bitched at Evan for things that Evan really had no control over, the employees that had the habitual Friday or Monday diarrhea, the last-minute scrambling to cover jobs because they just didn't want to show up. All of this I felt led to Evan's death and the more I thought about it the more it made me hate that place! Those that had always been there for Evan, I'd only wish them the best, but there was no way I could keep this albatross around my neck.

As I fumed, I continued to blame everyone and became even angrier at the world! I called Sarah and told her to let the employees know I will no longer be operating the business. We will be shutting down in two weeks, buy new padlocks so we can start locking the place down. Sarah was almost stuttering as she responded, "Mallory, you can't do this, Evan would never want the business to be shut down, you have both worked so hard to bring it to where it is." I didn't care. I was not listening; I gave Sarah every valid reason to shut the doors.

"Mallory, I want you to take some time, I'll run the business, I want to be here, I know this is what Evan would have wanted. Please just let me give it a try." I honestly had faith in Sarah, she had been the office manager for so long, I know that Sarah could do it, I just needed to change my mindset. "Sarah, do you realize that place killed Evan? I'm going to give this three month, if it doesn't work out, then we are going to do it my way!"

I wanted everyone that ever did Evan wrong, to now pay the price. In my mind they were partially responsible for Evan's death! I knew there would be slugs that would want to show up at Evan's funeral, I did not want them there! I called every one of them, "Don't bother showing up for Evan's services, you couldn't honor him while he was living, don't bother trying now! You did everything to attempt to destroy him and his business!" I called my sister in-law Karen that had put us through hell for years "I don't want to see your face at Evan's funeral!" I was on the warpath, and God forbid if any of these people tried to reason with me! I was wound up so tight, walking with blinders, not listening to any rational human being. They were all enemies in my eyes!

Our long-time family attorney was working around the clock so that I could gain access to our business accounts, pay bills, and make payroll. He was jumping through hoops with the banks because Evan had no master plan in case of his untimely death. I was at a point where I had no access to the business finances. The turnaround time was crazy, the amount of paperwork required to release funds was ridiculous. It seemed like every time I met with the banks, they were once again requesting a copy of Evan's death certificate. I finally lost it one day in the bank, I had a check to deposit, but it was issued to me and Evan, and the teller handed it back to me, and said "I'm sorry you can't deposit that without Mr. Mills signature." I grabbed the check and loudly responded "My husband passed away a month ago.", her response "We will need a copy of the death certificate before we can process the deposit." "I have given your bank three copies of Evan's death certificate to date, this is complete bullshit that you don't have it here on file, I'm so sick of this fucking run around!" At that point the manager arrived by my side and walked me into his office. I was having a complete meltdown; I feel I'm losing the battle. After a good half hour in the bank manager's office, I'm calm and ready to leave. The bank manager assures me that going forward, they will have Evan's death certificate on file. I apologize to the teller as I leave, I feel horrible, I've lost it in public, and now I'm apologizing, I just want to go home! I've turned into a Monster!

My day had only gotten worse when our family attorney called to tell me, "Mallory, due to Evans death, and Bryan being a minor, Bryan would be a Ward of the State until I had been found to be fully competent enough to care for my child. That does not mean Bryan will be removed from your home, he is appointed a guardian, you will be interviewed and evaluated by the guardian." I responded, "What the Holy Fuck does this mean, I am competent!" "Mallory, please calm down. This is standard in a case when a spouse dies. Everything is going to be all right; you have nothing to worry about, it's the safety and welfare of the child that must be followed up on." I thought, "oh my god I just lost it at the bank. Will they know about that, will they think I'm not capable of raising Bryan?"

It seemed like every little comment made; I was taking it personally. I recall Hailey asking if she could sell the 4-wheeler that her dad bought her. She no longer rode it, and she didn't want to see it in the garage anymore, my response like a lunatic "Holy shit Hailey, let's start selling everything, let the neighborhood think we have to have a fire sale now that your father is gone!" It was personal. All of it was personal to me. I was watching our home and family like it was a fortress. I did not want anyone to know what we were dealing with on a personal and emotional level as a family. I did not want them to assume that we were finally crumbling. Hell, a lot of them would have been applauding!

It reminded me of a comment that my sister-in-law Karen used often, generally if she got wind of some rumor we weren't doing well with the business, she would say, "has the princess finally fallen from her pedestal?" Her words echoed in my head. I felt like she was the enemy that never made Evan's life any easier. Anything she could do to throw a monkey wrench into our lives, she would be all over it.

I wanted things in our lives to settle down before we started making decisions to sell anything. I didn't want the slugs and the

Karen's at our doorsteps like vampires drooling for a little tidbit. The part I wanted to control the most, was showing Bryan that nothing has changed, our lives were still normal.

God, in my head I knew it wasn't normal, but for my kids I was trying with all I had to make it that way. As I'm saying this, I look over at Bryan, he is at the kitchen table still working on that whale project for school. I looked at him, "Bryan I thought you were all done with that." Bryan looks at me, "Mom, I'm giving him mean eyes." I think to myself, is this his normal right now, is this his distraction to what is really going on in our lives? I can't deal with Evan's death. I can't sit down and have a conversation with Bryan about his dad without crying. His silent pain is killing me!

THE CAVE DWELLER

To say the best place for me after Evan passed was in a cave may sound kind of nutty, but I think it would have helped! I did not have the desire to interact with other people. To sit with someone and have a conversation was like listening in an echo chamber. I would stare, hear garble, and shake my head up and down in acknowledgement. I couldn't hear them; I couldn't comprehend what they were trying to say to me. I don't think my mind wanted me to stuff anything else in my brain that would require thinking. I would leave a conversation never really knowing what I was just told.

I would go to the office almost every day to meet with my sister in-law Sarah. As soon as I opened the door the familiar smell of Evan's work shirts would hit me. My ears would begin ringing and my anxiety level would shoot through the roof. I would quickly make my way into Sarah's office and sit. The office, the desk once had been Evan's. The pictures that hung on the wall had all been gifts I had gotten him. The wooden coat rack in the corner still held his favorite caps. I was there to be brought up to speed on what was going on with the business, half the time I was off in another world.

The employees in the office would stop in and make idle chit chat. I know they felt just as uncomfortable as I did. It was difficult to look at them, I felt their pain and sorrow. I know they were hurting and grieving, and still were showing up to work. I on the other hand, despised this place! Evan lived and breathed this place. I would finish what I needed with Sarah and leave.

I would hurry back home. I would never turn the television on, I wanted complete silence. My brain was struggling to deal with the little information that it was already taking in. I had the hardest time remembering to do things. I would write them down and still forget. I guess that may have been my way of not acknowledging things or not allowing them to take up space in my head. So many times, I would hear the term "Widow brain", the fogginess and disconnect after the loss of a spouse. It was my brains way of helping me cope, to shield me from the pain and significant loss of Evan. What it was doing was creating a complete cluster fuck to my days!

I would keep the lights off when I was alone. I swear I could almost hear the electricity humming when they were turned on. My ears would pick up the slightest sound. My senses were on high alert. I would go around the house and turn all the ringers on the phone so low that I could not hear them. The only way I would know we had a call was by the sound of the answering machine going off.

The meals I would eat, would consist of toast, water, and coffee. I had no appetite, and eating, just never came to my mind. It appears I could eat one meal a day and not think about eating again. I recall my weight had plummeted by 30 pounds within six months. My clothes would hang off my body, I would grab a belt and a long shirt to hide the fact that I was getting so thin.

I would avoid having any company, I sometimes would sit in my house and watch my neighbor pull in, knowing full well I was not opening that door. I would respond to very few people if they called or sent a text message. Typically, it was the ones that I knew would break down my door or call the police if they did not hear from me. The ones that I was close with understood it was very difficult for me to function. At times things just felt like a hurricane and a wasp nest exploding in my head, the frenzy of it all turned me into a limp zombie.

The numbness in my body left me not giving a shit, I did not care about myself. I would leave my house without combing my hair, sometimes wearing the same clothes that I had worn the day before. I felt if I obliged to what my mind wanted, I'd be mentally okay that day. If I began to shower, try to do my hair, and get my clothes out I began to feel completely overwhelmed. I knew if I got to the point of feeling overwhelmed my anxiety would kick in and I would be back on the couch staring at a wall all day in the dark.

I felt I was broken, that life for me would never be the same again. The broken merchandise that would live its life out on a sales rack. So many would pick it up, admire it and think it could be just so pretty, if only! To see them set it down again and know that it had lost all its original sparkle!

I knew I could quickly transition to almost human when I heard my son's school bus pull up to our driveway. I would quickly turn on the television, race to the dining room and turn on the light. I know that each day it was my children keeping me alive. I witnessed this every time I heard their voice or seen their face. I could overcome anything for them!

I know this is part of my healing, it will not be pretty, and it certainly will not be peaceful.

TIDES OF CHANGE

Our home was quiet. The craziness began to simmer down after Evan's funeral. I wanted to focus on Bryan and Hailey, I wanted to be present in their lives again. The last three weeks were life changing for all of us. Our first evening of sitting down and having dinner as a family was difficult. The kids were silent, they barely touched their food, it all felt very forced as we set our emotions aside. Bryan left the table early. He wanted to go back to school. He was like me, burying his emotions, distracting from the ever-present elephant in the room. Hailey found solace in Noah, holding back her emotions until she left our home.

Bryan has stayed home for the past two weeks. He wanted to go back to school. He wanted to see his friends. On the car ride into school, I'm asking Bryan "are you sure you want to go back to school, you can stay home longer you know." I wasn't sure if I was saying this more for him or me at that time. "No, mom, I want to go back to school." We arrived at his school and began unloading the box carrying his Humpback whale project. I watched Bryan walk into school, his long strides keeping him a few steps ahead of me. It's today, we will see how everything goes for him and for me. We've been attached at the hip for weeks. I gave Bryan a hug and watched him stroll up the hall along with the whale that had endured with us, some of the worst days of our lives.

Hailey has graduated from college and started a full-time position; Noah was back to work as well. Today, it's me, the dogs and the four walls, at least until noon and then back to school for Bryans school fair. I finally got the phone call from the court appointed guardian for Bryan, my attorney was right, it was not as bad as I had thought. I was worried about nothing and could finally rest easy that Bryan was safe with me.

After dropping Bryan off at school, I stopped at the grocery store, I couldn't remember the last time I had actually went out grocery shopping, but the cabinets were getting bare. I rolled the shopping cart down the aisle, avoiding eye contact with anyone coming my way, hoping that anyone I knew was at work! I made my way to the coffee aisle, I had always loved the smell of fresh coffee brewing, and lately, I found myself brewing it just for the aroma. "Mallory, hi, I'm so sorry to hear of Evans passing. How are you, how are the kids?" This is exactly what I was trying to avoid, it was the parent of one of Hailey's classmates from high school. I looked at her and gave her a half smile, and kept on walking, I knew she meant well. It just was not going to go well in the coffee aisle. I grabbed my bag of coffee and headed to the checkout as quickly as I could.

    I kept thinking of the question I had just been asked, "how are you and the kids?" How does the outside world see our family? Do we appear to be okay? I feel like we're under a microscope being scrutinized as others look at us with pity. I didn't want to think about it, I preferred to avoid people and their questions. I did not remember much of my drive home from the grocery store, all I could think about was my encounter with Hailey's friend's mom, and the answers that I could have given her. I opened the garage door and pulled my car in, I took a sigh of relief as I heard the garage door close, knowing that now I was protected from the outside world. I grabbed the bags from the car and headed into the house.

    I pulled the coffee out of the bag and opened it, I put my nose to the opening and breathed in deeply. The aroma was something I always smelled as I walked down the hallway in the morning. At times Evan was up before me, sitting in the living room watching the news. He would hear me and smile as I approached.

    Today I grabbed a coffee filter and started a fresh pot; I rinsed the old coffee from my coffee cup. I sat at the kitchen table and watched the steam slowly rising from the coffee maker. If I closed my eyes and took in the aroma of the coffee I could picture Evan in his chair, waiting for me to join him, his smile always got me, not a care in the world when it was the two of us. My daydreaming had to end for now, I had to get back to school for Bryans class fair and the unveiling of "The Humpback Whale!"

RESISTING CHANGE WILL BREAK YOU!

    The mere thought of Evan's clean clothing sitting on our dresser gave me comfort. In my mind, I felt that he just did not have time to put his laundry away. The dark blue t-shirts and workpants neatly folded, the socks and underwear in their own separate pile nearby. I would leave these clothes sitting there for months on end, thinking again that Evan may be coming home. My mind kept telling me over and over "Mallory, he just hasn't put any of his things away, leave them be!" I would agree with my mind once again.

    Every night, every morning, my mind would start, "Mallory, keep telling yourself this, he will be home!" I would eventually have to agree. I just know it will happen. His toothbrush is still resting in its holder in the bathroom. The robe he just wore hangs from the rear of the bathroom door. His slippers are still next to our bed. There is still the faint smell of his cologne in our bedroom. The phone charger that he has misplaced so many times sits draped across his nightstand. His heavy work boots sit at the front door, just waiting for him to slip them on and head to work.

    My mind had one mission, the same message over and over in my head "leave everything as it is, don't change anything, if you change anything you're going to lose everything you knew of Evan!" That fear of thinking I would lose everything frighten me so much that I was afraid to change my routine. I would get up every day and follow the same exact routine.

    I would walk down the hall; I could smell the freshly brewed coffee. I would grab my coffee cup and fill it. I would sit at the table looking out the dining room window, watching the birds. I would chuckle remembering Evan saying, "Mallory, we are way too young to be watching the birds, isn't that something the older people do at the park?" I would always wish for a cardinal to show up, knowing that this would be a sign that Evan was visiting me. Most of the time it was just the pain in the ass squirrels visiting, they would have climbed the tree and dumped most of the seed to the ground. I guess I couldn't get that pissed at them, all the dumped seeds did eventually bring some beautiful cardinals to visit.

I would soon hear rustling coming from Bryans bedroom. I knew that at any minute he would be dragging himself out to the living room. Bryan had the same routine in the morning. He would flop on the living room couch, grab the blanket near him, wrap himself up, and curl up into a ball on the couch. I would turn on the television and start making him some breakfast as he watched his favorite cartoon.

The only sound you could hear in the home was the silly laughter coming from the television. Bryan would be sitting there staring into outer space at the television, eating his breakfast with half a smirk on his face. At times I was not sure if Bryan was smirking because of what he was watching or what he was thinking. Did he wake up every day wishing for the same thing as I did? Did he sit and wonder about the same things I did?

For us, it was just going through the motions of just getting by each day. We were keeping it simple, with no crazy changes, sticking to our routine.

Once I got Bryan off to school, it was time to push myself to get going. I was working at a local medical facility finishing my college internship. Today was the day I would attempt to go again! I had been telling my supervisor for weeks that I would be back, and he was always so kind, saying "Mallory, take your time. You're always welcome back when the time is right."

I was enjoying my internship and learning so much every day, this was something that I looked forward to prior to Evan's passing. I had hopes of picking up my internship where I had left off once I felt strong enough to go back. It is not that I did not try, there were so many days I would get in my car, prepared to head to the office but would end up frozen in fear. I would sit in my car and think "Mallory, you can do this, Mallory dammit, just do it already!" Every morning it was the same outcome. I would get in my car, do the whole encouraging speech, sit defeated and cry. I fucking hated myself. I thought I was weak and useless! I was afraid to step outside of my safety bubble.

The faces I had seen on a regular basis at the medical facility would be expecting the same old Mallory, confident, smiling, outgoing and happy. This was not the Mallory today; they did not want to be around this new Mallory. The new Mallory was anxious, afraid, withdrawn, emotional and not up for socializing. My outside began to match my inside, Ugly! Sometimes I would go days without showering or combing my hair. There was no putting on a happy social face for eight hours a day.

I am not exactly sure how many attempts I made or how many weeks I had been doing this routine. I sat in my car and realized, I needed to text my supervisor and end the internship. The game I played daily was not helping anyone. It was not fair to the medical facility to continue to hold my internship when in reality we all knew how this would end.

I never did end up going back to the medical facility where I was completing my internship. After Evan passed, I knew I was not mentally nor emotionally prepared to deal with people. Me going back at this time was not going to happen!

I had finally decided that my main and only focus at this time would be my kids. I would stop trying to push myself to be somewhere that I knew my mental state was not going to allow. I would keep the daily routines as close to the same as they had always been. I started having Hailey and Noah over for dinner just like in old times. I wanted to keep things as they always were. To accept change would be accepting the reality of life without Evan.

Every day things were going good with my mind and mental state. I would stay in the house, do my everyday routine, chores, prepare dinner and invite the kids over. We would sit together after dinner and talk or watch a movie as a family. At times we would sit with Bryan at the kitchen table and help him with his homework. It was all working perfectly. I thought this may be the new normal that we had talked about, its finally happening.

The days and months passed; the weather began to get chilly in upstate NY. I remember being at the grocery store picking up supplies to make one of our favorite winter comfort foods, chicken, and biscuits. I put the chicken in a large pot of boiling water and started mixing the biscuits. All the delicious aromas in the kitchen, reminded me of so many chilly winter nights when we stayed in and just snuggled under a blanket and watched movies. It was a good idea to make popcorn and do just that tonight with the kids!

Noah had arrived a little early for dinner, he sat down in the kitchen and had a cup of coffee. Noah popped the lid off the chicken and biscuits, "One of my favorites. I can't wait for dinner." We talked about this evening and having him, and Hailey stay longer to watch a movie with us. "I'll even break out the popcorn maker and make it an official movie night tonight!"

I peeled the remaining meat off the chicken and tossed the bones in a bag. I knew I would be sorry in the morning if that bag of chicken bones stayed in the house all night. I grabbed the full bag of chicken bones and headed outside to throw the bag in the garbage can. As I turned the corner at the garage, I seen Evan's truck. I immediately thought how great it was to have Evan home early from work and how happy he would be to see one of his favorite meals prepared. I thought how nice it was that tonight we would all be together to have dinner as a family. I smiled as this image ran through my mind.

I quickly ran back into the house; I knew I would find Evan peering into the pot of Chicken and Biscuits. I was happy and looking forward to seeing Evan. I opened the door and walked back to the kitchen. I looked at Noah, "Where is Evan?" Noah was quiet for a moment and said "Who, what?" I repeated, "Where is Evan, his truck is in the driveway, I just seen it!" As I was saying this, Noah just looked at me without saying a word. His expression was of hurt and confusion. "Mallory, are you okay? Evan is not here." My ears were ringing, I felt so hot I thought I would pass out.

I knew exactly at that moment that my brain was playing a very cruel joke on me. I stood in the kitchen with my mouth wide open, I was in total disbelief I had thought Evan was home. My heart was shattered, for that split second, I thought my world was once again whole. I was scared for myself and what control my brain had over my actions. All day I had been reliving the past, everything, it all seemed so real to me!

The happy remembrance of days like this and our favorite meal triggered my mind, that nothing had changed. I looked at the place settings on the table, I had even put a plate out for Evan! As much as my brain was attempting to protect me from trauma, it also sent me spiraling back to the worst days of my life!

I knew after this incident that it was time to accept all the things that I had buried. I thought by acting and pretending like things were normal and not changing anything I would be okay. My days were a planned routine to keep me safe and not deal with real life. The protective bubble I had been hiding in exploded today.

ACCEPTING CHANGE

I continued to struggle with accepting the change in our lives and dealing with Evans death. I was now going to face this head-on. No more head games! My brain just would not allow me to stop all the feelings of would have, could have, should have. They constantly swirled in my mind. It reminded me of being a child and hearing the repetitive click, click, click as the baseball cards hit the spokes of the bicycle tire, accompanied by the constant whizzing sound of the tires. It was repetitive, over, and over, my mind was constantly spinning. I would start to think that my brain was ready to move onto another thought, but no, it was right back to that same thought, click, click, click, the whizzing, the spinning. I could not get a thought straight in my head.

My brain was insistent that I was to think about every moment in those last days with Evan and ask myself what I could have done differently. Maybe if I had taken Evan to another hospital to manage acute care, we would have had a better outcome. Then I would say "No, Mallory, Evan was dealing with the flu, any hospital was capable of dealing with the flu!" Taking him to that local hospital for the flu should not have resulted in him dying. They should have been able to treat Evan for that!

I could have argued with Evan, I could have been adamant that he was going to the larger, better equipped hospital. What the hell, Evan wasn't feeling well, I wasn't going to start an argument with him at that time! Again, I felt he just needed fluids, he was dehydrated and not acting like himself. Who knows, maybe it was the Codeine in his cough medicine that was making him slightly delusional.

This process would go on and on in my mind constantly. At night I would lay awake thinking over and over what I could have done differently to save Evan. I lay awake at night thinking about the people that had wronged Evan, made a shamble of his life. They made so many attempts at complicating his business that he was spending a lot of time putting out fires and not focusing on his health. I lay awake angry at the people that could have made Evans life easier, but instead they continued to stab him in the back and support those that were hell bent on destroying his business! I did know this, Evan's kindness, generosity and care of others was something that never changed, he was just a decent person, even to those that were assholes!

The eyes of his family, my children, his employees, and our community, all looking at me as though I could have done so much more to save him. The pleading with the doctors and the angry outbursts with the medical staff. I was blaming all of them when in reality I blamed myself for not being able to save him! How in the hell could I even attempt a life at being normal when I carried so much guilt. I felt I could have done so much more to keep Evan alive. God help me get through this! How could I have let this man die?

So many nights I sat by Evans hospital bed, hoping for the slightest eye movement. I was wishing he would squeeze my hand to let me know that he was going to turn things around, and that he was going to make it through this. There were times when I would talk to him about our children, thinking that this would be the moment that he would respond. I could clearly visualize him screaming at God "I'm not dying. I have to live for my wife and children!" As the days in the hospital dragged on, I pulled every trick out of my hat, searching for something that would trigger Evan's mind and bring him back to us. We needed a miracle, and we needed it now!

I was dealing with the fear of the unknown and a million hurdles that I did not know if I had the strength or the willpower to be able to make it over them. The thought of me raising my kids without their father felt like a hard kick to the stomach. The anxiety attacks felt like my heart was going to beat out of my chest and I was going to die! I would still sit in the parking lot at a scheduled appointment and end up cancelling it. I just could not do it! Every possible fear was raising its ugly head. I knew I had to face my fears, but I was going to do everything in my power to hide this from my children. I felt this time that I could do it.

I know that I had felt in my heart that I could continue to live my life as though Evan was still here with us. Pretending and lying to myself had made it easier, or so I thought. I wanted to celebrate everything that Evan loved. I wanted to continue the traditions in our family that he always looked forward to. I wanted to enjoy all of this with our children and family. If there was something we celebrated in the past, I wanted it to continue in our household!

I wanted my kids to continue to feel the excitement of every holiday that we had celebrated in the past. I wanted our home to feel alive with laughter and the love that they had always known. I wanted this so badly!

Memorial Day was the first event that we celebrated without Evan. This was our first get-together after Evan had passed. I kept telling myself, we were not deviating from all our planned family events "you're doing this, Mallory!" The more I thought about not holding the party, the more I would hear Evans voice telling me to keep the family traditions going. It was important for a family to be together. I also felt this would be an opportunity for the kids to enjoy their family.

I so desperately wanted it to be like old times. I wanted Evan to finally show up, walking in like he had just gotten back from out of town. I knew this was not going to happen. I felt I finally had my brain in control. I felt in the past, the delusions began to happen when I got deeply involved in reliving old memories and not focused on the here and now. Today's get together may be what our family needed. I just wanted to be reassured I was making the best decision by having the party with family. We had all been dealing with grief and I was hoping bringing everyone together would help us heal.

In the past, we would have a big family barbeque. The pool would be open with lounge chairs sprawled all over the deck. The coolers are loaded with cold drinks and the meats marinating in the fridge. Every time we planned a party, Evan joking would say, "Hey Mallory, make sure we have enough food. Remember that wedding?" "Evan, you tell me, you tell everyone about that wedding, how could I ever forget." In the past Evan had always talked about a disastrous wedding he once attended. The establishment ran out of food, and they were unable to feed all the guests. An argument ensued between the bride's family and the venue. He would say, "Mallory, come on, can you imagine that happening." I would reply, "No, Evan, I can't. That's not something you want to remember about your wedding day." So, from that point on any party we were planning, Evan always made it a point to jokingly remind me of that wedding.

Between Evan's large family and mine, combined, we had some of the best parties. Throw in a handful of good friends and the laughs, drinks, and tasty food. The fun never seemed to end. The kids would be running back and forth between the pool to the jungle gym, screaming and playing. At dusk, everyone rounded up their kids, said their goodbyes, and off they went until our next get-together.

The next day would be just as comical as family and friends posted their pictures on social media. The pictures and the comments would have us laughing years later when these memories popped back up. They certainly bring me right back to that day. I would stare at those pictures and smile, knowing how fortunate we were to have such good friends and family to share our life with.

As much as I loved our family get togethers, I had not seen nor spoken to my brother Scott and his wife Karen in years. There was a falling out over a business venture we had together. Evan decided to go off on his own, thinking it would be best for the family and everyone else involved. As our business continued to grow and become more successful, we began to endure hateful verbal attacks against us. To maintain the peace at our family get-togethers, I decided it was best that Scott and Karen not attend these family events at our home.

Like clockwork, after our family get-together, Karen would begin her hate-filled text messages to me, saying I was selfish and ungrateful for not inviting them. I wanted so badly to respond to her, letting her know all the reasons they were not invited. This had been going on for over five years, and I just wanted it to end. Evan was completely against me saying anything because he thought that since they were family, "Mallory, they will come around, time heals all wounds."

It really hurt seeing my relationship with Scott destroyed. How did Scott sit by at times and allow Karen to do this to our family? The connection I had with Scott had always been close when we were growing up. I had thought of him as a role model. He was someone I trusted and looked up to in my adolescent years. He was the person that gave me away at my wedding. It was just too difficult to even think he was aware of what she was doing and allowed it to happen.

Karen would go to any lengths to show her hatred towards anyone that she was jealous of. One thing I'll never forget is the day I heard that she had asked my mother, "Where is the princess today." Karen loved to call me princess. My mother said, "Mallory is flying to Florida today with Bryan." Karen with no hesitation replied, "I hope their plane crashes!"

I confronted my mother, and she acknowledged that the incident did occur and said, "Mallory, you know how Karen is, she may have been drinking when she said that." I was horrified. I would never ever say this about my worst enemy, let alone their innocent child!" If this had been me in the car and this was my child referenced, I may have ended up in jail. I was pissed at my mother for not sticking up for me and her grandchild. To give Karen a pass for saying that and blaming it on alcohol pissed me off even more!

I would never forget this event as long as I lived. I knew Karen was evil, but I never imagined she was this evil. I knew at that time the shit with her would continue to the day Evan and I died, her jealousy and hate that we were successful burned her up inside. This recent event ended it all. I knew our relationship could never be mended. I knew going forward that I would never have anything to do with Karen or my brother Scott ever again.

The first Christmas without Evan was extremely rough for me and the kids. It hit us the hardest out of all the holidays. Evan always wanted the Christmas tree up the day after Thanksgiving. If he had it his way, he would keep it up until June. This was by far his favorite holiday of them all. We loved getting up and watching the kids open their gifts. Evan always wanted to open his gifts last. He would sit and watch the kids as they excitedly opened their gifts, just sitting there smiling ear-to-ear as he took it all in.

As difficult as Christmas was, in my mind, I needed to keep those memories alive as much as I could. I wanted this Christmas to feel like it always had when Evan was alive. I invited all our family and close friends. I made some of Evans favorite foods and played our silly games as Christmas music softly played in the background. We all laughed and shared some of our favorite memories of Evan. I loved watching my kids, smiling, and laughing with my family. This is all I wanted to see; I wanted to see them smile and not cry on this holiday.

I think as much as I struggled to have the Christmas party, I was so happy that we did. I swear Evan had joined us that night in spirit. I could feel that same calm and strength that he gave me in his presence. I think that night was the first time in many months that I was able to fall asleep without tossing and turning. I was slowly accepting Evans passing. It was now okay to talk about him and continue some of his favorite traditions without the crazy mind games.

The next morning, I woke feeling so refreshed. The tension that I had been feeling in my head and neck for months seemed to have subsided. As I walked out to the kitchen to grab a cup of coffee, I told myself that it was going to be a good day. I sat down on the couch with my coffee and started looking at the social media posts from family and friends and smiled as I went through the pictures and videos. I was so happy we could enjoy this Christmas together. I looked over at Bryan as he was putting together one of the new Lego sets that he received from a family member and, for that one split second, it felt like old times.

I thanked God for that moment. I thanked our family members that had been there and supported us through everything. I finally thought that I might have a chance and it was the best feeling in the world!

I was quickly brought back to the real world when I heard the dinging of my cell phone. It was a text message from Karen. Since I hadn't heard from her in over a year, it could only be one thing. She was ready to give it to me! I took a sip of my coffee and prepared myself for the barrage of anger and profanity. I knew that Karen had been up early, trolling every social media site, hoping to find something so that she could start the texts rolling. I knew from the past that she always tried to engage me to get me going, and I wasn't going there. I wouldn't give her the power to put me in a bad place emotionally! I opened her text message, "What a piece of shit. You are extremely inconsiderate!"

I responded back to her "God bless both of you. Have a good life." In my mind I thought that would be it and she would go away. At the very least I hoped that she would realize that this was our first Christmas without Evan and have a little sympathy and compassion. I set my phone down to go to the kitchen and pour another cup of coffee. I kept telling myself over and over "let it go Mallory today isn't the day for this!"

I heard the phone go off in the living room, another heartfelt message from Karen. "Fuck you and have a terrible life. You deserve it!"

I walked down the hall to my bedroom as all the past miserable memories of dealing with her after every Christmas came flooding back. Evan's insistent "let it go" in my ear. This time, I knew in my heart that Evan would not be okay with letting it go! I decided that I was no longer going to tolerate Karen's abuse. I sent a message to her children. "Please work with your mother, I'm not putting up with this any longer. If she continues, I'm calling the police."

My niece quickly responded, apologizing for her mother's behavior, and said she would call her mom right away.

The barrage of text messages continued from Karen; she was irate and possibly embarrassed that her children were now aware of what she had been doing to our family for years. I ignored her messages and called my neighbor and good friend Lexie. Lexie answered in a panicked voice. "Hey, Mallory! What's going on? Is everything all right? Are the kids, okay?" I responded quickly to calm Lexie, "Yes, we're all okay. Hey Lexie, would it be okay if you picked Bryan up and brought him over to your house for a couple of hours? I'm having issues with Karen again. I think it's time to end this once and for all and call the cops!"

Lexie was more than aware of the drama and hate-filled text messages that Karen had sent, me through the years Without hesitation, she responded, "I'll be there in 5 minutes!" As Lexie pulled into the driveway, I grabbed Bryans jacket, "Hey buddy, do you want to go over to Colby's house for a little while? I have to run out and do a few errands." With a huge smile, Bryan slipped his arms into his winter jacket and ran out the door and hopped into Lexie's car.

As I watched Lexie's car pull away, I knew tonight would be the last time I'd ever have to deal with Karen again! I was no longer going to put up with the abuse from Karen. Evan was no longer here to tell me to keep the peace with the family! The bullshit we had put up with for so many years, and it was always Evan saying, "Let it go, Mallory, their family." I would respond, "If this is what family does to one another, I'd rather hang with my enemies."

At this time, whether Karen knew it or not, she was chiseling away at what very little sanity I had left. Over the past few months, I had worked hard on my emotional and mental state, but today was challenging me beyond my limits. I was done with her bullshit. Enough was enough!

I picked up the phone to call the State Police and said out loud to myself, "Mallory, is this really worth it?" Damn right it is, I am done! "911, what is your emergency?" As the State Trooper walked up the sidewalk to my home, I'm sure he felt that this was just another domestic family squabble during the holidays. As he approached, I could tell he was around my age, late 40's or early 50's, A seasoned officer that had seen and heard it all during the holidays.

"Good evening, I am officer Dennick. What seems to be the problem? Our dispatch reported that someone is harassing you via text messages."

Oh boy, I felt the emotions and tears beginning to bubble to the surface, and I knew this was not going to be easy. The words came out of my mouth like a tossed salad of information, "My husband passed away this year. This is our first Christmas without him. Normally, I would never call the police, but this has been going on for years. My husband always stopped me from reporting it. I had to send my son to my neighbors so he wouldn't hear or see this." I have no idea how much officers Dennick caught as I rambled on through the tears and the sobs.

"Okay, okay. Have a seat and try to calm down. Now, who is this that has been texting you? Do you have the text that you can show me?" I pulled my phone out and brought up all the text messages from years past and present. I felt like such an idiot as I watched officer Dennick read the messages. Why did I let this go on for so long, and why didn't Evan just let me report this years ago?

As officer Dennick scrolled through the text messages, I could see that he was shaking his head. I could tell that he was not taking this lightly. "Excuse me for a moment, Mrs. Mills. I need to go to my patrol car and make a call. I'll be back in a minute."

As officer Dennick left my house, it felt like a huge brick had been lifted from my chest. I'd taken a stand to protect myself and my children from this ongoing abuse and harassment from Karen. It ends tonight! I watched from my living room window as officer Dennick talked with someone. Hopefully, he had reached Karen and told her the games had ended tonight.

Soon after, I see officer Dennick walking back up the walkway to the house. "Mrs. Mills, who is Noah?" I must have given him a really strange look, "Noah is my daughters fiancé. Why?" "Mrs. Mills When I called Karen, she proceeded to call me Noah, told me that I needed to fuck off, and proceeded to hang up on me. At this time, I'm going to pay her a visit at her home and let her know that if this continues, she will be charged with harassment. If she texts you again, I want you to report it immediately. Tomorrow morning, I will need you to go to the local State Troopers Barracks to provide them with the printed text messages, as well as a written statement regarding all the details of the harassment."

I walked officer Dennick out to his car. "Officer Dennick, thank you for all your help tonight. I know this should have been reported years ago, but my husband always wanted to keep the peace in the family." He just looked at me, smiled and said, "it sounds like your husband had a lot of patience and love for his family,"

As I watched officer Dennick pull away, I sent a text to Lexie. "All should be good here from now on. I'll be over shortly!" I smiled as I drove to Lexie's house. This was really the end of it. No more harassment from Karen. Amen! Ding Dong the Wicked Witch is Dead!

I sat in Lexie's driveway, waiting for Bryan to come out. As soon as I saw his smiling face, all the drama from earlier in the day just melted away. "Mom, it was so much fun at Colby's house. He got these cool Nerf guns. We built forts and ate popcorn." I smiled at Bryan. Such innocence is still inside this young man. I wished that I could bottle up that happiness for him to use in years to come. "I am glad you got to spend time with Colby, it was a really busy night, but I got so much accomplished. I think tonight we should go home, have ice cream and watch movies." Bryan looked at me and gave me two thumbs up.

Now I could see that it really was a good day for both of us. I had the strength to deal with Karen today, to finally end it all, and it felt good! I don't think Karen would ever see beyond all her jealousy. All the good Evan had done for her and her family while trying to keep the peace fell on death ears.

Tonight, I looked back and thought how quickly they forgot, that years ago Evan paid their company's back Sales Tax which at the time was over a hundred thousand dollars. Ironic huh? Evan was trying to help save their business as they were still hell-bent on destroying him and his business. I guess it's true when they say, "No good deed goes unpunished."

If Karen had only realized that, for all these years, nothing was done because Evan wanted peace in the family. Not only for our family but for hers as well. I knew that Evan was cheering in heaven, knowing that my choice tonight was for our family's peace. This change in our lives felt great!

SOCIAL HAUNTING

The months passed and the New Year was approaching. Bryan and I spent New Year's Eve with my sister Payton and her family. A community event was being held. We spent the evening watching Ice sculptures being made and a brilliant display of fireworks at the end of the night. During the entire evening I watched couples walking hand and hand and strolling through the streets with their children. I could hear them laughing and singing along with the local bands as they played. I knew that every one of them was proclaiming how grateful that a New Year was upon us, new life adventures awaited us all.

I hadn't felt the old emotions in so long I was scared when I felt the anger, sorrow and grief grip me that evening. I wanted what they had! I wanted Bryan to walk around and laugh, throw snowballs, and have hot chocolate with a man that he could look up to. I wanted someone that I felt safe with, someone that I could carry on an adult conversation with. I just wanted to try and move forward, even if it was a little bit. The events of the past year always creeped back into my head, the tick, tick, tick of the baseball card in the bicycle spokes, the never-ending swirling of memories. I felt I could never escape the traumatic events of my life! I forever would be that angry person, jealous of what everyone else had, constantly comparing my life to theirs.

I had seen and felt this anger before, I'd had remembered a moment in my mother-in-law's kitchen soon after my father-in-law had passed. I had been standing by the kitchen sink, I heard this loud banging on the dining room table. I turned to see my mother-in-law slamming her small frail fist into the dining room table. She was crying and shaking her fist, yelling at the sky, "damn you, Earl, damn you, why, why?" I could see her pain, the tears rolling down her cheeks, and I could hear her anger at this man that left her too soon. I can now understand her anger. We felt betrayed and lonely. We had lost our loyal protector, the one we would love forever.

That evening I lay in bed, I couldn't shake the anger and jealousy I felt towards all the happy families that gathered that evening for the New Year's Eve event. These feeling were becoming common again. This is how I felt I was ending the evening after every social event that I had attended! I always put up a good front at these events, but when it became intolerable, I'd just leave. It got to the point that I was making excuses not to go or just not showing up after saying I'd be there.

I felt comfortable with Payton. She was the one that I opened up to with everything going on in my life. She experienced it firsthand with me after we all went hiking together one day. The hike was great. Bryan was enjoying himself, and the fresh air and beautiful mountaintop views were amazing. I remember taking a deep breath and taking in a huge swallow of air. Payton waved to me and said, "smile!" I look at that picture still to this day. That woman in the picture is broken. She is thin, frail, and weak. The eyes are sunk in, rimmed with a gray shadow. I'm just there, with no emotion and no effort in that smile, I hate to look at that picture, I hurt for that woman, I can feel her pain and grief.

We made our way back down the mountain and headed to dinner at a local favorite restaurant in the area. As soon as I walked in it hit me, the families sitting at the tables, men with their arms around their wives, and the kids battling for airtime with their parents. I hate them! Again, there was no reason for me to hate them. It was plain and simple. They had what I once had!

We were finally seated at our table, and my brother-in-law Brent started talking about what a good day we had. They were laughing and smiling. At that moment, I felt I was on the outside looking in. My mind was taking in everything, all the families smiling, all the laughter. I got up from the table and went into the restroom, and burst into tears. I felt so sad for Bryan. He would never have this again. My heart was breaking not only for me but for him as well. Evan was a very affectionate dad, if he were here, his arm would have been around Bryan or me.

I pulled myself together and went back to join everyone at the table, Bryan was busy doodling on the menu with the crayons that they had given him. He was in his own little world, quiet, looking down and coloring. I often wondered if he was struggling with everything around him, as well. Did he have the same emotional breakdown seeing kids with their dads? I put my arm around him, as he looked up, he smiled at me, I knew at that moment that this was something that he needed. I knew I had to be strong for Bryan. I knew I had to work on my issues of anger and bitterness toward other families. I knew that I had to live a happy, stable life for him and Hailey!

I felt with this New Year I needed a positive change in my life, I needed to be able to be the old me! As with every night, I lay in bed talking to Evan, asking him to give me the strength to be a better, stronger person. I wanted reassurance from Evan that in the New Year it was going to be okay to begin to move forward, to begin to enjoy life, to get out and socialize and have fun! I said "Evan, please send me a sign that life is to be lived while we are still here on earth."

HAPPY NEW YEAR

I had the most beautiful dream last night; I woke up and immediately wrote it down so that I would not forget. I was dressed in a white ball gown, white satin shoes, my hair pulled up, and I looked as if I was preparing for my wedding. The room was completely pure white in color, the walls, floors, curtains, everything white! I could hear the music begin to play, a soft violin and piano, something you would hear in an elegant restaurant. I heard footsteps and turned around to see Evan. He was wearing a black tuxedo. I took his face in my hands and said, "I knew you would be back; I've missed you so much." Evan never said a word. He held me as we waltzed around the room. It was so strange because neither of us knew how to Waltz, but we had discussed taking classes for Hailey's wedding. Was this the dance that we never got to enjoy together? My God, this feeling was like pure heaven!

Our celebration was interrupted. It was my nephew, Daniel. He was across the room calling out to Evan. I watched Evan turn to look at Daniel, his arms slowly releasing me. I screamed, "Evan, no, you are not leaving me! Daniel, what are you doing, why are you taking Evan!" I was screaming so loudly; my voice was vibrating off the walls. Evan did not look back at me once, Daniel just kept saying, "Evan, it's time to go." I was pulling Evan's arm with all my strength to keep him with me. The way Evan was gracefully walking away was effortless, it was as though Daniel was a magnet.

The room suddenly got quiet. The walls appeared to have water flowing down them, the reflection from the water made it look like crystals sparkling off the walls. The floors were now covered in water, again it appeared as though I was standing in a room so brightly lit by the reflection of all the crystals. Was this my souls visit to Heaven? Was this my goodbye to Evan that I never had a chance to do? I never wanted to ever forget this dream or all the emotions and feelings that I had during it.

I could not wait to call my sister-in-law Sarah and tell her about my dream. It was her son Daniel in my dream with Evan. "Sarah, I've got to tell you about the dream I had last night!" I spent the next 10 minutes going over my dream with Sarah. "Sarah, what do you think this all means? It has to have a meaning behind it?" "Mallory, maybe it's to a new beginning. Maybe it was Evan letting you know he is okay; it could have so many meanings." "You're right. Maybe I shouldn't look into it too much, it will make me crazy, but I absolutely loved the dream, it seemed so real, like Evan was really there with me."

The phoneline became silent for a moment, "Sarah, are you still there?" "Yes, I am, I received some bad news this morning." "Sarah, what's going on, is everything okay, did someone get hurt?" "Mallory, Greg passed away in his sleep during the night, I got a call this morning." I thought the air had been sucked out of the room, what, why, how did this happen? Greg was the young son of Evan's cousin; he was in his early twenties. This young man was in the prime of his life and just like that he was gone, I could not wrap my head around what I was hearing. I thought of Greg's family, his mom and dad, and the pain that they were dealing with, it was awful news. This poor family, I could feel their pain.

I felt that I had been angry and bitter for the past year, and with each moment that I spent being pissed off at the world I was robbing my children of their happiness. How could they be happy when their mother is a robot, acting as though all is good in the world, hiding the fact that she was still in denial, playing make believe? I knew after that dream, and the tragic news that I had heard today, that it was time to move forward, embrace life and enjoy my kids and family. I knew the only way that I was going to do this was to begin seeing a therapist. I needed someone that was unbiased, someone that knew nothing of my life. I loved my family and friends and appreciated that they were looking out for me, but each one of them had a different opinion on how I should be living my life.

THE SUN THROUGH THE CLOUDS

On Tuesday morning, I got Bryan off to school and focused on finding a therapist. My first approach was to reach out to my primary care physician for any recommendations. Next of course I began to search on social media. I had worked in the medical field for eight years, and the exposure to what happens behind the scenes made me look a little closer at the qualities I wanted in a therapist. I knew that she had to be a female, someone that could relate to the typical day-to-day struggles of a mom and wife. I did not want someone that was just listening to me talk, I wanted someone that would set goals and expect me to achieve them.

After a thorough search I found a therapist that I felt checked off all the boxes on my wish list. I nervously called the office and scheduled my first-ever appointment with a therapist. The relief I felt knowing that I would be sitting down with someone that would help guide me, get me through some of my darkest day. To help me work through the anger, jealousy and bitterness that kept rearing its ugly head.

On the day of my scheduled appointment it was lightly snowing, I got Bryan ready for school waited at the end of our driveway with the car heat set at high. This had been our first Winter without Evan. There was so many things Evan handled, plowing the driveway, shoveling the sidewalk, taking care of the furnace. I knew my concerns would be quickly put to rest with all the help from Noah, my brothers, and brother in-laws. I was so fortunate to have a big family as well as married into a big family, everyone was ready to step in and help in any way that they could.

The school bus arrived, and Bryan hopped out of the car and off to school he went, waving as he ran up the stairs on the bus. Again, I was so fortunate to have a caring compassionate son, always so concerned of others, quick to give me a great big hug as soon as he walked in the door after school. If this young man only knew how many times, he had brightened my day, my problems were nothing when I see his smiling face. Of course, Hailey was a strong supportive force, she was such a responsible adult, our conversations turned to encouragement, and willingness to help each other through our daily struggles.

I pulled out of our driveway, and as I drove, I thought, "what do I tell this woman? What information do I keep to myself? What do I want to share with her?" The questions and concerns began to swirl in my mind, "what if I tell her something and she judges me poorly? Will she think I'm a bad mom because of how I've felt at times?" The more I scrutinized what I was going to freely share, the more I realized that if I were not honest, if I held back, if I lied, I would only be hurting myself and I would never find healing.

I pulled into the parking lot, a large red brick building looming before me. The double doors in the front with frost at the corners, concrete stairs covered lightly in snow, iron-rails, it all looked cold and unwelcoming! I did not want to get out of my car, I thought for a split second of turning the key in the ignition and going back home! "Okay, Mallory, get your shit together, stop making excuses, get in there!" In a huffy agitated manner, I grabbed my purse and car keys, I swung the car door open, the frigid wind hit my face as if to say, "turn back." I slowly made my way up the concrete stairs and walked through the glass door. A sign on the right directed all patients to check-in with the receptionist. As I walked into the waiting room, I could hear trickling water. As I looked around, I could see a small water fountain in the corner. The sound of white noise buzzed in the room. I sat down and closed my eyes. All the sounds in the room put my stress and anxiety at ease.

I was startled by the receptionist as she lightly tapped me on the shoulder, "Mallory, hi, Samantha is ready for you. Please follow me." As I followed the receptionist down the hallway, I noticed the signage on the door I was entering, Samantha Styles. LPC. As I entered the room, I noticed it had the same relaxing feel as the waiting room. In the corner was a fireplace, the flickering flames and heat were so welcoming. The entire exterior wall was all windows. The warm sun was shining through, lively plants were placed all around.

I sat down on the couch, and the immediate image that flooded my mind was of someone lying down on the couch, was I supposed to do this? I preferred to sit down; I may fall asleep if I had laid down. I made myself comfortable on the light blue couch, as I nervously picked at my fingernails waiting for Ms. Styles to arrive. Every passing second, I sat waiting made me more and more anxious!

"Mallory, hi, I'm Sam, it's nice to meet you." My first impression of Sam, she was someone I knew I would have been good friends with, in the outside world. A genuine smile, minimal makeup, and a disposition that made me feel at ease. I always got concerned with people that overdid it with their makeup and clothes. It made me think of the old Mallory that struggled with her identity, and always felt I had to have a perfect image for others to approve of me. Basically, a superficial image! I knew Sam was confident in her skin. What I saw was what I got from this woman!

"Hi, Sam. It's good to finally meet you." "So, Mallory, please tell me a little bit about yourself. Take your time, and just tell me what you feel comfortable sharing at this time. I may have some questions as you go along if you don't mind. Of course, that's if you feel comfortable answering them."

I knew as soon as Evan's name left my mouth, our session would be all about me crying my eyes out. Sam was quiet the entire time. She let me pour out every bit of grief and hurt that I had bottled up for so many months. What I had shared with Sam was nothing that I had shared with any family or friends. It felt good to talk, not be judged or advised on what I should do. As much as I loved my family and friends, at times I felt what they were telling me, was what was good for their lifestyle not mine.

Sam looked over at me, I knew she was still absorbing all the information I had just fed to her in a matter of minutes. "Mallory, why do you feel you carry so much guilt with what happened to Evan?"

Sam's question made me angry! I replied, "why wouldn't I feel so much guilt? I could have done so much more, I could have demanded his primary doctor see him again, I could have made Evan go to a hospital that was more equipped to handle his level of care that he needed, I could have screamed louder at the nurses and doctors handling his care!"

Sam looked at me and asked, "Mallory, would Evan have allowed you to do this? What would he have wanted?" "Dammit, I knew Evan, and I knew that he would have wanted to go wherever it was the most convenient, and quickest. Evan did not want to be sitting in a waiting room waiting for his primary to prescribe him something else for the flu. Evan would not have wanted to go to a large hospital to sit in a crowded waiting room. He wanted quick in-and-out service!" Anything that delayed him or interrupted his workflow with the business was out of the question!

"Mallory, you can carry this guilt for the rest of your life, but clearly you were acting on what Evan wanted. Do you think if he were standing here today, he would have changed anything?" I knew Evan would never have changed anything, but me, yes, I would have done things my way. Evan was so stubborn; he would not have changed a thing! I remember a moment in the hospital thinking how pissed Evan would have been when he woke from his induced coma. He would be spitting nails seeing that I had him admitted to the hospital. I was honestly stressing about this the entire time in the hospital, this was a decision I had made to have him admitted. The physical and mental state that Evan was in led me to no other choice, I felt what I was doing was the right choice.

Sam was right, and I was right there giving her the answers that I already knew. There was not a chance Evan would have allowed me to admit him to the hospital, or take him to another hospital, or scream at the top of my lungs in anger at all the hospital staff. That just was not the way Evan rolled. Evan was a lowkey humble guy, who would say "handle it", no matter how or what it took, to get the job done in the quickest, calmest manner!

We did just that, we went to the small community hospital! At that point, his body was reacting to Sepsis, which again we were under the assumption that Evan had the flu. We did not need a big city hospital, right? That was my guilt, which would be the cross I had to bear my entire life! A thousand times I said, "if only I had taken him to a level one trauma center, he would still be alive!" My brain would quickly remind me, "but Mallory, we were dealing with the flu!" It didn't matter it was a constant cycle of guilt in my mind that just never gave up.

I continue to tell Sam, the doctors voice in my head repeating, "Sepsis in its very early stage has similar symptoms as the flu, fever, fatigue, and body aches." Those symptoms I reeled out to the front desk receptionist on intake, "he has the flu, I think he's dehydrated, he just needs fluids." Those words playback in my mind, repeatedly. "Sam, I had so many opportunities to make it better."

The last time I actually spoke with Evan coherently was outside of the Emergency room. After completing his intake paperwork, we stepped outside to get fresh air. I remember he looked, so pale, so weak. He had no strength to stand and asked if I'd get him a wheelchair. It wasn't long after that that they were bringing him to a room to be evaluated. Evans health quickly declined in the hospital after he was admitted.

These events and moments are burned in my mind. I looked at Sam and said, "As right as you are this is the toughest hurdle to overcome. The one thing, I regret not being adamant about is the hospital he chose to go to!"

"Mallory, you did everything that you possibly could have done on that day, you never knew exactly what you were dealing with, until it was beyond your control." Again, Sam was right, we followed our primary care doctor's orders, took the scripts, and waited for improved results. it just never happened; in hindsight, we now know why. I had no idea how long Evan had the infection; I only know that during those two weeks of treating the flu with antibiotics, he was not getting any better.

As Sam raddled off questions, I felt comfortable and openly answered them. And then Sam asked, "Mallory, at any time did you think about suicide?" I stopped for a moment before I responded to

Sam. I could lie and deny like the old Mallory and respond as though I was tough and strong. I could act like I totally had my shit together and say the thought never crossed my mind, or I could continue to be honest.

"It wasn't that I wasn't depressed at times and felt so lonely, but I'd never take my own life. Though, I do remember driving, I was alone at the time, and a semi-truck was approaching from the other direction, I knew at that moment if he had crossed into my lane, I would not have tried to avoid him."

I think I shocked myself by revealing this information to Sam, but I knew I had to be honest. I can look back now and realize that it was a dark period in my life. If not for my kids, things may have not turned out the way that they did.

It's not easy to talk about depression or suicide but it's there, you can attempt to hide it from others but it's there! I would look in the mirror and wonder who this woman was. I had lost 30 pounds, and the dark circles under my eyes told the world that I barely slept. The grays in my hair had seemed to pop out overnight. My body at that time was running on anxiety, fear and coffee. My appetite consisted of pushing food around my plate and nibbling occasionally.

As much as my family raised their concerns, I always told them that I was fine. I always felt I could handle my emotional state on my own and would never need the help of a therapist. It was clear to others by looking at me that it would benefit me to make that phone call and scheduling an appointment. It took me a year, but I'm thankful that I finally took their advice and reached out to Sam.

My session with Sam was an hour long. When I walked out of her office that day I was emotionally and mentally exhausted! It felt good, though, all the months of lying to myself being in denial, and playing make believe on every level, was mentally and physically exhausting! I know I have a long road ahead of me, and several more sessions of therapy, but this is a step in the right direction. My plan on healing and moving forward would be an hour session every two weeks, or until I got this evil monkey off my back. I looked forward to my next session with Sam, she helped breakdown a lot of the walls I had put up.

You may not want to hear this, but it is something I deal with often. You will not have your "normal" again in life, because with that comes great memories. Those memories bring back happy moments, those happy moments always bring us to the one key factor, our loved one that is no longer here. Grief is a vicious cycle, and it will consume you if you allow it. The anger, fear and anxiety will put you right back in mental and emotional lockdown. To avoid catapulting back down that dark mountain I focus on all the "new normals" in life. All that I should be grateful for, and not hateful for what I had lost in life.

I would silently thank Sam for helping me through so much. If I had never reached out to her, I would still be frozen in fear and never able to move forward in life.

A COMPANION DOES NOT MEAN I'M LOOKING FOR SEX!

As the months past I continued to deal with the anger and jealousy of seeing happy families, this holiday, that holiday, the vacations, the smiling faces....blahhhhh! I thought it would become bearable at some point. The constant reminder of something that we would never have again, or would we? I found this was a topic that Sam and I often discussed in therapy.

I think one of the hardest things for someone to do after the death of their spouse is to move forward in life. The moving forward part is not only difficult for you, but your children, your family, and your in-laws. There is no written rule that says, now is the time to begin to live your life. No rule that says, go have dinner with a companion, or now is the time to go catch a movie, or go for a walk. This part of life did not come with a handbook. There are so many difficult hurdles, and this was one of them.

You are constantly questioning yourself and feeling the guilt of even having the thought cross your mind. How dare you to even consider that selfish thought! Do you honestly think you deserve to laugh and be happy again! What a fucking whore, your husband died, now you want to have dinner with someone! Do you know what your husband went through and now you just want to forget it ever happened! This vicious cycle is never ending, those voices screaming in your head, telling you how horrible of a person you are. That moment you were so close to saying yes, quickly followed by guilt, sadness, and sorrow. You crawl back into your nutshell and hibernate that selfish thought away. Again, you pray for light at the end of the tunnel, and you ask God to give you strength to make the right decision.

In my session with Sam, I brought up the "Companion" subject. "Sam, it just does not feel right, it's almost like I am attempting to replace Evan." "Mallory, there is no rule book in life. What do you think Evan would want for you in life? Would Evan want you to grieve for him every day, or would he want you to try and move forward in life and be happy? Mallory, if the tables were turned, what would you have wanted for Evan?"

I knew the answer to all of Sam's questions, Evan and I had covered all these topics. We had so many family and close friends that had passed, it was inevitable that this topic would eventually come up. We did have our rules and recommendations for each other, depending on who went first. We wanted the other to be happy, we wanted someone that would love our kids as if they were their own. We wanted someone that would provide a stable and supportive home life. We knew this person whomever it was, would be a huge presence in our kids' lives. Neither of us were big drinker nor partyers, of course that someone had to meet all these criteria as well.

If I was ever to do this, I wanted someone that did not know me, someone that would not feel sorry for the poor widow. I needed to bring someone into my life that would make me laugh, laugh so hard that I cried. Someone to have a conversation with that did not involve the trauma that I was dealing with. Someone that someday may understand that I was damaged goods, mentally, and emotionally unstable at times! This to me sounded like a lot to ask for.

In my head I felt the one thing that always held me back, was that I was a widow. I have no idea how I'd react to going out, no matter how innocent it was. I felt I had baggage, I had a hard time socializing, I had a hard time seeing people happy, I felt guilt at the thought of laughing and having a good time, I cried easily. The list went on and on. I think I'd throw someone into a complete depression before the evening was over!

I would lay in bed at night and think of Bryan not having a dad or a role model. Bryan was still young, he always talked about Colby and his dad and the things they did together. It hurt me to see Bryan longing for what his good friend had and all the fun they had together. It was easy for me to become angry and jealous as Bryan talked about them! As much as I tried to fill Evans shoes, there were just some things as a mom I was not good at. I tried the fishing thing, which after several attempts at putting a worm on a hook without gagging, I had to give up. I had gotten Bryan involved in so many sports and activities, but it just was not the same. The parents on the sidelines killed me every time! I wanted to sit on the sidelines and be left alone. They knew us and knew our story. I always wondered if Bryan was also finding it hard to fit in like me. If Bryans heart wasn't into whatever activity, it was, I just let him quit!

I just wanted us to be accepted without judgment!

I did not want Bryan to grow up without someone that he could look up to, someone that would teach him to be a great man. A person that would give him the tools in life to be a confident young man. A man that he could go to with any question there was in life and feel he was going to get an honest answer. A man that would lift him up on his darkest days. A man that would love him like he was his own.

I would go to Sam with the same question every other week, "Sam, how do people move forward in their life after losing a spouse?" It was an emotional roller coaster to even begin to think of it, it just didn't seem worth it at times. Then, it would happen again, Bryan talking about Colby and his dad doing stuff together, all the parents at the sporting events rooting their kids on, family outings. It never ended, a daily smack in the face. I would leave my therapy appointment thinking, "this is the week I'm going to move forward!"

The guilt I carried for my children was horrible. I almost felt responsible for their sadness. I always felt that in some ways I could be doing more. I could somehow distract them from the reality of life, making them smile more, laughing, and carefree again! Something that seemed so easy was so fucking hard!

Could I bring someone into our lives to help us, help me. That certainly would be a tall order to fill.

JUST COFFEE

After months of going back and forth to therapy I mentioned to Sam, "I think I may be ready to meet someone for coffee." "Mallory, that's a huge step for you. Remember, just go on your terms if you don't feel right excuse yourself and leave. This is a big hurdle for you, I don't expect it to be easy. Keep it short and simple and see how it goes. This will be a slow process for you."

Meeting Eric for the first time, I chose to meet at a coffee shop that was in a nearby city. As I sat in the parking lot, I felt incredibly nauseous, I knew it was my nerves. I sat in my car and composed myself, taking deep breaths to calm myself down. I looked at my watch, it was 11:05, I was late. I summoned up the courage and opened my car door and headed to the coffee shop. As I walked, my legs felt like Jell-O. My supportive voice came in my head, just as it had so many times before as I sat in the garage trying to go to work. "Mallory, you can do this!"

I walked in, I looked around for Eric. I glanced over and saw him sitting at a table. Eric looked nothing like Evan, blonde hair, stocky build, and a bit shorter. I wanted it that way. I did not in any way want to feel that I was looking at a mirror image of Evan or attempting to find a man that look exactly like him. This man would be a companion, a friend that I could meet for coffee, dinner, or a movie. Maybe at some point we could take Bryan fishing or catch a basketball game. My brain quickly interrupted my thoughts, "Slow down Mallory, we're not there yet!"

I waved from across the room, Eric got up from the table and approached me. "Mallory, hi, I didn't think you were going to show up." I looked at Eric, smiled and said, "I didn't think so either." I instantly noticed the smell of his cologne it was nothing like Evans, that warm, woodsy smell. God how I missed that smell! We sat down and ordered coffee and discussed what he did for a living, his family and some of his hobbies. I kept my answers very generic, not wanting to disclose too much information to a man I hardly knew or even knew if

I'd see again. One moment in my head, I'm thinking this is great and the next is, I'm not sure if I'll ever do this again!

We started discussing some of the great comedy movies we had seen over the years. There was an instant when we both laughed about the same scene in a movie, it broke the ice and for the next twenty minutes we just talked. Eric and I were both on the same page, we were not looking for a relationship, we were just interested in a companion to go out with occasionally. This would work out perfect, I could safely test the waters, get myself acclimated to society once again, and have a quiet dinner with some quality adult conversation. We kept it at an easy quick half hour, I thought I could do this again!

I looked forward to my meeting with Sam the following week, I had so much to fill her in on after my meeting with Eric.

OUR DAILY PEP TALKS.

Ever since Evan had passed, I found myself carrying on a daily conversation with him. I'd be driving and know that spiritually he was in fact, a passenger in my car. Today was no different than any other day, I would be talking out loud, hand gestures and all. As cars drove by, they would look in my direction with a confused looks. I would continue with my conversation without a care in the world. Any questions that I had, any situations that were bothering me, came up during these drives. Do I think this helped? Most definitely, it gave me a sense of peace freely talking with him.

I had kept Evan's cell phone, safely tucked away on my nightstand. I had dragged his charger to my side of the bed to keep the battery charged. I would sit in bed at night and go through all the text messages that we had sent one another. I would look at the funny pictures he had saved on his phone and smile. One of the images was at the beach. It was our last Anniversary that we had celebrated together. We stood with huge cheeky smiles standing in front of the Lighthouse in Maine. If I looked closely, I could see the smear of cocktail sauce on his shirt from dinner earlier in the day. I remember the moment that cocktail smear occurred, the shrimp cocktail at dinner!

That weekend get-away with Evan was remarkable! In the early morning walking the beach with a cup of coffee, dinner at our favorite restaurant and finishing the night off with drinks by a crackling fire.

The long drive to Maine was no bother to us, we talked endlessly. We stopped to grab coffee bright and early in the morning and off we went. This day, we were in no rush, just taking our time. We stopped halfway to have lunch in Boston, and back on the road to Maine. We would arrive in Maine and do a little shopping at the outlets, we had to make sure we bought something for the kids. The kids were not happy that they were not going on this trip, it was an adult only weekend! I'll never forget that weekend, it was the best time that we had in a long time. Evan was relaxed and really enjoyed his time away from the office.

I missed the sound of Evans voice. I would listen to the messages that Evan had left me on my cell phone, over and over again. Evan's strong authoritative masculine voice saying, "I love you. Hi, just calling to check on you and the kids. I hope your day is going well." There were days I thanked God that I still had these messages to listen to, it helped me in so many ways to hear him say, "I love you."

Many nights before going to bed I would grab his bathrobe and wrap my body up in it. I'd close my eyes and smell his cologne. I'd envision him lying next to me once again. I would pray that evening that I would have a dream about him, to see him, to talk with him. I would wake the following morning feeling like I had not slept at all, disappointed that not once during the night did, I dream about him.

I did not think at any time that this was strange or odd. This was my way of holding onto what little I had left of Evan. I never felt that me doing this made me look crazy. This little ritual of talking in the car, reading old text, and listening to old voicemails gave me strength. I knew I would always have a guardian angel by my side at all times. I felt Evan's presence around me wherever I went, I knew I was protected by him, as well as our children.

As I got in the car today, the conversation with Evan started. "Evan today was a day that I felt I could attempt to move forward. It was difficult today meeting Eric, he definitely is not you. Today I actually laughed and enjoyed a conversation with a man other than you. I don't know if I'm going to be able to do this again. The guilt is now crushing me!" I sat quietly, praying for a response. I just wanted back that part of my soul that I was missing!

As I lifted my head, I saw a truck pull into the parking spot in front of me, the sticker on the rear window boldly screaming Evan's favorite football team, the Dallas Cowboys! I have always been very spiritual, believing in Angels and Spirit guides. I was going to take this as a sign that Evan heard me, and acknowledged he was okay with me moving forward in life. Honestly, I did not need a sign, I know Evan wanted me and our kids to be happy in life no matter what it took to get there.

The emotions of allowing someone new in your life was like opening the windows in the morning. You could either get the warm sunshine with a beautiful breeze or a gloomy day with a cold breeze. Emotionally I could feel exactly how my day was going as soon as I opened my eyes. That mood always impacted my days and how I dealt with others. You could get the warm sunshiny Mallory, happy and ready to socialize, or the cold gloomy Mallory that was anti-social with the covers over her head. It's very difficult, the emotions are different every day, it would not be easy for an outsider to understand.

CROSSING THAT BRIDGE

My newfound companion made me laugh and smile again. Moments with him interrupted my brain and my constant thoughts of losing Evan. I wasn't looking to forget Evan, I wanted to retrigger my brain to know once again what it was like to smile and laugh. I began to look forward to going out to dinner or the movies with him. I had forgotten how comforting it was to have an adult conversation. I continued seeing my companion, we were still both in agreement that we were not ready for a serious relationship.

My family and friends were finding it very difficult to accept the fact that I was going out with a man. I know it hurts them. I'm sure in their minds they felt that I had completely betrayed Evan. There would never be a chance of that ever happening. It was important to me that my companion was aware of Evan, and the significant place he still had in my heart. I knew from the get-go that whoever came into my life would have to be accepting of me as a widow, my children, and the love I still had for Evan.

As I continued to see my companion, my relationship with some of my family and friends deteriorated. The ones that had been there during some of my darkest moments were now talking about me behind my back. In my eyes I felt what I was doing was very innocent. I could not understand why they would not want to see me happy again. I honestly felt that I was at a turning point in my life. The days had been dark and heavy for so long! To me it was like I had clawed my way out of a cold dark well and seen the warm sun shining for the first time!

The few family members and friends that still called and hung out with me, either accepted the fact that I was going out or accepted it the best that they could. We would meet up for dinner and one evening went out to listen to a band. The events of that evening and some pictures that Lexie posted on social media turned into a nightmare! One family member saw the post, did a screen shot and sent it to the other one. An immature tactic, but this one family member, definitely the pot-stirrer of the family!

I woke the following morning with a text from Susan, "You are a fucking whore, how can you do this to my brother!" I had no clue what Susan was talking about because I hadn't even been awake long enough to see what the hell she was talking about! A few seconds later it was the picture Lexie had posted, I called her and asked her to remove it. "Mallory, why? There is nothing wrong with that picture!" "Lexie, just remove it, you know how the family feels about things." "Mallory, how did Susan even see this picture, she is not on social media?" "Lexie, I'll give you one guess." Lexie, responded, "Never mind, that explains it all?"

So, the text messages from Susan started at 8:00 a.m. and continued up until 7:00 p.m. that evening. "You are an embarrassment to this family. You and your retarded friends think you're all thirty years old!" All this coming from Ms. Morals who two years prior was so upset with Evan and a business proposition with Brady that she told Evan "I wish you would die!" Her habitual angry always got the best of her. So instead of living my life how Susan felt I should be living it, I blocked her number and have never spoken with her since. I felt there is nothing wrong with shedding old relationships as you grow and change in life!

I first noticed the disconnect between family and friends when I was no longer getting phone calls or text messages from them. Then I started to notice that we were no longer invited to the parties at their homes. I would throw a party and ask them if they wanted to attend, I wouldn't get a response, and they wouldn't show up. For me it was no longer a question of them being upset with me, I knew the answer. What bothered me the most is that Bryan was also being dragged into the mess, he was no longer getting invites to any parties.

It was a year later, and Susan threw a 70th birthday party for our sister in-law Penny. I was talking to Hailey and happened to ask her what her plans were for the day. This is when I found out about the birthday party. I was pissed because once again, this is Bryan's family also, why wasn't he invited! I could give two shits about going but don't hold our differences over Bryans head also. The conversation between Hailey and I had gotten heated. I ended the call saying, "Bryan doesn't need them anyways, and hung up."

    I would go on with life, as would Bryan. When Bryan became an adult, he could decide at that point if he wanted them in his life. I was not fighting anymore battles with the family. To me, this was all petty. Life was too short to continue fighting with this family. I decided before anymore crap was seen on social media, I would distance myself from them, out of sight out of mind! I wanted peace in our life, and this was far from it!

    Over the years, things have mended between me and many of my family and friends. I wish at that time they could have understood what I was going through.
I'm much stronger now and I'm in a better place both, mentally and emotionally in life. That does not mean that I don't think of Evan every single day and from time to time still have emotional breakdowns. I know that now I have a very good support group that I can rely on.

    I know that someday we all must experience death and grief. I dread the thought of any of my family or friends losing their spouse. I don't wish for any of them to deal with the pain and hurt that me and my children did. What I do know is, if this every happened to them, I would be by their side supporting them all the way.

    I look forward to my days with my kids and grandkids. I thank the Lord every day for helping me get this far in life. I must give my therapist some of that credit as well! Her words not mine, "You may occasionally disappoint others but make sure to never disappoint yourself." I'm grateful to my Lord that he has let me live yet another day and I know someday I will be with Evan again.

Don't wait for everything to be perfect before you decide to enjoy your life.

-Joyce Meyer

BUILDING A NEW WALL

In life you will always find you have your cheerleaders; you will also find most people that want nothing more than to see you fail. Your happiness will only bring sorrow to them. Your sadness will brighten their days.

The time after losing Evan I always thought I could depend on my closest friends and family members to support me. Of course, this all changed with the addition of the "companion." I can understand that they were all hurt, for them to see so much of my life transitioning away from the life that I had had with Evan. I wanted so much to move forward; it had been the toughest years of our lives. It certainly had shown me the true colors of certain individuals. I'll never regret the people that I had removed from my life for the darkest times when I needed them most, they were hell set on breaking me down. In my mind I always knew that Evan would have been so disgusted with the way that certain individuals treated me and our kids.

I am now a much more confident person; I am strong and I'm resilient! I don't allow anyone to pass judgment on my life or my children's. I don't tolerate them disrespecting me or my kids, they have no right or no say in what goes on in my life or in my kids. I have done a damn good job of crawling out of the ashes and raising my children. I don't feel I ever have to answer to anyone, my business is my business! In my life, I want peace and if you can't bring that to my life you will no longer be a part of it! I owe no one an explanation for the decisions I've made or the things I've done in life.

I love my children and I am grateful that I have them and that's all I need in my life! Your opinion means nothing, going forward I wanted to have a life of happiness. I wanted to see my children smile again I want so much for Bryan to have a male presence in his life. I wanted him to have those moments in the garage where you have those typical questions that only a man could answer "how much air do I put in the tire? When do I check the oil level." I wanted nothing more than a positive male role model for him.

The pain and the judgement I felt when bringing someone new into my life almost destroyed my life. My relationship with so many family members and friends ended! I know so many of them had their own thoughts and feelings on how I should live my life, but I also feel none of them knew how much pain they were inflicting on us. I wish for only one moment for one day that they would wake up and experience what me and my children had been through. I was as strong as I could be on days, but this was only for my children. I didn't care what these people thought of me!

I had made the decision that going forward I would only do what was best for me and for my kids. Fuck them if they didn't like it! I had set up boundaries and not one of them would ever break that boundary. I expected them to respect not only me but my children. I wanted peace, and if you did not bring that to my life, you would no longer be a part of it. I wanted to be happy again.

I know that Evan would have only wanted support from our family and friends after he left this earth. I know that Evan would have wanted to see us happy, to move forward. I know that he would want my children, especially Bryan to have a positive role model in his life. The emotional turmoil that all of us were dealing with was difficult. For anyone to sign up for this had to truly be a strong person I respected. That person came into our lives. He gave us the stability to move forward. He is a role model for Bryan, and an exceptional Papa to Hailey's children.

If you ever are in a position to help a grieving friend or family member, give them all the support that you have because there will be times when they wished it were their last day on earth. I don't think anyone of my friends or family looked at me this way because I hid my pain so well. This was only because I thought I had to be so strong for my children. Denying my pain was only destroying me inside. All these years that Bryan and Hailey struggled, not one person seen their pain or felt the grief that they were dealing with. It was always about how they expected us to live our life. The constant expectation fed into their ears made them feel that supporting my decisions in life was wrong. It created so much confusion for them on who was right and who was wrong.

    As you go forward in life always remember your departed loved ones will always be by your side. Take the time to talk to them as though they are right there. Do not for one moment give a fuck about the people that want to judge you and the decisions that you make! For as difficult as life is, I know you're trying to climb that mountain to reach that top, to see that sun shining and dance once again! The anchors in your life, let them settle to the bottom of the sea, move forward, and live your best life ever!

FINDING YOUR SQUAD

I knew that if I was going to change myself, I really needed to change my mindset!

I started focusing on my daily routines again, which one of them was to make dinner every night. I loved to cook and giving Evan a healthy homecooked meal every night had been important. This man was up and out of the house by 6:00 a.m. every day, he deserved a good meal when he got home. I knew I was no longer cooking for Evan, but the portions did not seem to change.

I would cook way too much food for Bryan and me, and by the end of the week, I'd have tubber-ware bowls spilling out of my refrigerator. I had recently read about a local group on social media that helped the homeless. This could be a solution which benefited me and the organization that supported the homeless. I figured I would continue to cook as I always had, and all the extras would be donated to this group. In my eyes, this was a win-win situation.

I reached out to Myia; she was the founder of the organization I had read about. I told her I thought what she was doing was fantastic, and how grateful I was to see her so involved with the homeless community. Myia and I decided to meet at her home Thursday evening to find out how I could become more involved with her organization.

With crockpot in hand filled with, you got it, home-made chicken noodle soup, I headed out to Myia's house. I think we all have a vision in our heads of a person prior to meeting them, but mine was spot on! I rang the doorbell, and the loud barking of dogs followed. Soon after a young lady in her early 30's answered the door, "Hi, you must be Mallory. Come in." Myia was like this totally cool chick, like an earth child, with tattoos, neat jewelry, ripped jeans and a t-shirt, a totally authentic person. I knew we would become great friends!

Myia explained that she had started the organization after her dad had passed away that year. She wanted to find a distraction from all the pain she felt from her father's death. I felt completely the same way, ever since Evan had passed, I knew I needed a "distraction" from my daily life, something that would give me a purpose in a positive way, and this would be it!

So it began, every Friday night I'd bring all the extra food to Myia's house, she would prep it all, preparing it into small containers. I stayed busy cooking everything, and anything, knowing that what I was doing was helping a great cause. My mind was now focused on helping others, which meant cooking for Bryan and me, and adding extra for our Friday night meals for the homeless.

During all of this, I'm honestly not sure if Myia ever knew how much she helped me mentally, and emotionally. I had a purpose that would give me something to look forward to, and at the same time I was helping Myia with her dream of feeding the homeless.

As the months went on, I became more involved with Myia and her mission to help those in need. On hot summer days, we would take gallons of ice cream to the inner-city parks and hand out ice cream cones to anyone that wanted one. We planned a BBQ fundraiser and had an amazing turnout, raising much-needed funds for the cause. Any skill or talent that anyone had, they brought to the group to help Myia and her cause to help the homeless.

On a Friday night you would see a long line forming, of those in need waiting for a meal, hygiene products, or clothes. You name it, and the volunteers came through with it each week. Myia did not miss a beat in evolving her mission, every holiday, birthday, or special occasion was never missed for a child in need.

As the hot summers continued, we scheduled a night to provide haircuts. I gathered up my scissors, clippers and cape and made my way to the inner city park, where we met every Friday night. To me and to others a haircut is a haircut. We just walk into a salon, and we get it done. The homeless have less of an advantage; they don't have the financial means, and many salons are not that welcoming to the homeless. That night was an eye-opener, for women, and men that had not had their hair cut in months, or years, feeling great about themselves. To see the smiles and the gratitude was very heartwarming. This distraction was feeding my soul in a good way. It was bringing back the kinder, happier Mallory.

My mind was starting to shift its focus, the non-stop click, click, click of traumatic memories were not in the forefront of my mind any longer. The thought of helping others was comforting, it gave me the drive to do more to help out. If at any time I became idle, the memories crept back in my head. I'd quickly pull out a cookbook and start doing an inventory of ingredients and start cooking!

Life as we know it, tends to throw a monkey-wrench into things when it all is going well. I had been home watching a movie with Bryan, it was January, and it was bitter cold out. Bryan and I just wanted to stay in that night and avoid the cold. My cell phone rang, and it was my sister-in-law Sarah, it wasn't unusual for Sarah to call us and check in on how things were going, but normally not this late. Tonight, Sarah was calling to let me know that Evan's cousin Rob had passed away earlier that day. My heart sank for Rob's family, in every way, they were a tight-knit family, happy, caring, and loving. Rob, just like Evan was the matriarch of the family, always there for his family no matter what.

I couldn't stop thinking of Rob's daughter Jenn, she was older than Hailey, but she loved her dad the same way Hailey had loved her dad. When Hailey lost her dad the prior year, it shook her world. There was nothing that was going to take that heartache away. For a daughter to lose her dad is like taking away all that safety and security that she felt in the world. The phone calls about tire pressure, oil changes, and leaking faucets now seemed so overwhelming. Dad is the only one that had all the answers.

I remember months later I reached out to Jenn. "Hi, Jenn it's Mallory. I was wondering if you would like to go out to dinner Friday and then go listen to a band with Eric and me." "Mallory that sounds like fun. Do you mind if I bring a friend along?" "The more the merrier!" We went out that Friday night and had such a great time together. It was fun to let loose, dance and just listen to the band. I knew tonight would not be my last night I hung with Jenn. Together we laughed so much! That was the start of a great friendship!

Pretty soon it was Myia, Jenn and me hanging out. We would travel to the beach, go out to lunch, laugh until our bellies hurt. Our friendship was based on lifting one another up. There was one thing we all had in common. We all suffered the pain and hurt of losing a loved one. We knew the value of kindness and compassion. We all had lost someone that could never be replaced. Our lives never revolved around petty drama or materialistic values. We were all grateful for one another's support and knew how precious life was!

COMPARING APPLES TO ORANGES

A friend once said to me, "I can understand what you're dealing with. I lost my mom." I said, "Can you honestly understand what I'm dealing with? Do you wake up every morning and notice the other side of your bed is empty? Do you notice when the bills are piling up, and your mortgage is due? Do you still have another person you can depend on financially? Can you understand the loss of love and intimacy from your spouse?

It's a fine line when offering advice to someone that has lost a loved one. We should also never feel we are in a position to judge them unless we have experienced the same exact thing. Our grief and emotions are not the same when we lose someone that we love. Yes, we all feel pain and the heartache, but there is no way to compare one's suffering. The grief is so much different when you lose a spouse, child, sibling, or parent. The grief that you are dealing with is completely different from the grief that I am dealing with.

Can you understand the pain a child is going through at his sporting event when he looks to the sidelines and see's all the dads rooting their sons on? I can guarantee you that, in that game and all games going forward, his focus and attention will not be on the game, but on the one person missing from the sidelines. As the mom of children that lost their father, I am always trying to find the best way to deal with their pain and hurt. There are no substitutes for birthdays, graduations, or weddings. These celebratory moments will not be the same for my kids.

I remember going to my nephew's wedding. This was the first formal wedding I had attended since Evan had passed. It was a beautiful wedding, and I was so happy for my nephew. The entire evening changed for me when the bride walked onto the dance floor and began to dance with her father. It instantly changed my mood, those feelings of being so happy changed to sadness. As I watched others around me cry tears of joy and happiness, I was crying tears of grief and sadness. This was one of the hurdle's I had not yet experienced, I never thought I would have reacted this way. My first thought and feeling that ran through my mind was, Hailey never got to have that dance with her father. I felt over the years I had become so strong and was capable of handling anything. Time does not make it any easier!

That moment right there validated once again all the things in life that we would never get to experience with Evan. To some people it may sound odd, when I say, "Our loss is not the same." I can never relate to your loss, but your pain and your hurt, I can relate to that. My children have faced so many obstacles in life and dealt with so much after losing their father. I will say it a thousand times, our family's grief is not the same, but the pain that we feel for losing the one that we loved is there!

Our daughter Hailey did get married the following year after her father's passing. She stated in no way would she have a traditional wedding without her father to give her away. It was a destination wedding held at a beautiful Island resort. The day of her wedding I was struggling emotionally, I knew it would be hard but not like this! The old Mallory came out, the denier, the I'm okay liar! Hailey looked absolutely beautiful in her wedding dress. We sipped champagne and did a cheer to her dad in heaven before going out to the beach for the ceremony.

The music was queued, one of Evan's favorite songs began to play, "Somewhere Over the Rainbow." My heart sank, the pain in my heart I felt for Hailey not having her dad here was all over my face. I walked down the aisle and took my seat. I was suddenly angry with Evan, "Evan, why were you so stubborn, why didn't you go to the doctors when you needed. Why did you leave the hospital against medical advice? Dammit you should be here today for Hailey!

That day I continued to drink champagne until I was numb from all feelings and emotions. I was not a drinker, so it did not take a lot before I was no longer feeling the pain. I got so sick in the bathroom I almost missed the reception. Our friend Maria came in and got me and dragged me back to our hotel room. I remember her looking at me and saying, "You're going to lay down for a little while. After that get, your shit together! This is your daughter's wedding day and you're not going to miss it!" Maria was right, I needed to find the strength to deal with this and it certainly was not going to be with more champagne!

I was really upset with myself and felt guilty that I had almost ruined my daughter's wedding. I don't think that I can thank Maria enough for helping me that day. I needed her at that time more than she will ever know. The old Mallory needed her ass kicked and Maria was right there to do it. And as much as I hate putting this in my book it had to be said. The good times, bad times and the shameful moments where our demons come back full force. The pain of grief has no privacy exclusions, no timetable of when to arrive or leave. It can be the ruler in your world at any given time!

For those that have lost a loved one, I will never pass judgment. I will never tell you how to live your life. I will tell you to never stop loving yourself. I would tell you to accept the love and support of family and friends. I would also tell you to set strict boundaries with some family and friends. I think sometimes people see us as vulnerable. They feel they must step in and direct every decision in our lives. We begin to lose ourselves as we allow them to direct our decision and pass judgement on the decisions we make on our own.

Do not ever feel that seeking help from a therapist makes you appear weak. To seek out a therapist was one of the best decisions I could have ever made for myself and kids. There were times in my life when I felt my thoughts and emotions were going haywire. To sit down with the therapist and put everything out on the table helped me to clear my mind, it helped me to make better decisions in life.

Do not go into a therapist's office thinking, "I am tough, I am strong! I am going to go in as if I have my shit together." No, do not go in with your shit together! Let that shit spill out! Everything that you have been holding back, everything that you need to say, let it all come out! Over the years the worst thing I could have done to myself was to act like everything was normal and I had it together!

My shit was not together! It was a huge lie full of fear, immobilizing me from moving forward in life.

Live your dreams, not your fears!

MY HOPE IS TO LOVE YOU AGAIN!

It took me a real long time after Evan had passed to find me, the real me again. I had started slipping back into bad habits of feeling that materialistic things would make me happy again.

I had always been that poor girl growing up. There were times in my younger years we lived in homes with no heat or running water, dependent upon food stamps. As a child you don't see or feel the impact of not having necessities. If you weren't raised with this in your life, you simply did not miss them.

I think one of the hardest things about growing up poor is I developed this thick skin. I proclaimed to myself, "When I am older, no one will ever know that this girl right here was dirt poor, EVER!." Shallow, right? I was driven to bust my ass to make lots of money or at least enough to buy me whatever I wanted.

I become so superficial I forgot where I had come from. I bought all the best cars, homes, designer bags, and clothing. I would walk out of my home freshly made-up, not a hair out of place, even if I was headed to the grocery store! The ego has told you; this is the only way people will approve of you, "Keep that image on point. You don't want them to see that poor little girl!" And when ego spoke, I listened!

That ego will strut right along with you in the mall and tell you that you need that designer handbag, "Mallory, it will make you stand out amongst others! "Get it, Get it, Get it!" You will walk out of that mall feeling pretty dam confident, carrying that oh so ego desired bag. The weeks and months will go by, and the ego could care less about that expensive designer bag that had once given you that glimmer of happiness for a short period of time. The glimmer is gone. Ego is now ready to splurge again.

The shoes, clothes and handbags spilling out of your closet that you may have only used a handful of times, sit there waiting for their turn to be worn. They want to scream to the world "look at me, look at me, I am expensive, I am beautiful, aren't I? As we stare in our closet, we ask ourselves so many times "Why did I need that, why did I spend so much money on a dam bag?"

My ego would be quick to respond, "Mallory, do you want to look like Beth in those dowdy cheap clothes? Seriously, she doesn't even have that many friends! Or do you want to look like Savanah, a totally cool, hot chick, did I mention lots of friends! Mallory, please say Savanah! I don't think anything in her closet cost under five hundred dollars'! She always looks amazing!" Ego won again; I hated my ego!

If we felt that everything, we bought would make us happy forever, what a beautiful world we would live in. It is definitely not the case, we become conditioned to shop, as a want not a need. We begin to learn that when we do shop, it makes us feel good, look good, and ready to confidently take on the world. Superficial with a capital S! Take that money and start investing in YOU! Take that trip to the beach, book that massage!

Our ego protects us, which the widowed Mallory, really needed. It never wants us to remember that poor greasy haired girl, wearing the hand me downs, being teased on the playground. It wants us to keep on going in the direction it has taught us for years. That we too can have anything and everything, and it strongly encourages it! We will pass that legacy onto our children, only buying them the best name brand shoes and clothes. Secretly praying they will be invited to the most popular kids' parties!

And here I am, I'm that girl! I grew up with 4 older brothers and one older sister, raised by a single mom. I was 4 years old when my dad moved out and ultimately divorced my mom. Prior to this, we did have a good life, a home, food, and gifts on our birthdays and holidays. After my parents divorced, I would have given anything to be like Savanah in school. With the nice clothes and pretty hair, she had the perfect life, right? I would ride the school bus home and watch as kids got off the bus, thinking "wow, they have a beautiful home!"

Later I would see our stop, an old dilapidated two-bedroom trailer, no running water and a woodstove in the living room that provided heat. How I hated that walk of shame getting on and off the school bus each day.

I remember my older sister Payton, every Sunday at the laundromat with bags and bags of dirty laundry, with all of us younger kids trailing behind her. Thank God for Payton! She was like our second mom, doing our laundry, cooking our meals, and kicking our ass if we needed it. Payton had to have only been 15 years old herself, with so much responsibility thrust upon her at such a young age. Payton was mature and responsible for her age, I guess she really had no choice considering. I have no idea how she shouldered the burden of so much at such a young age. I had always been grateful that Payton was my older sister. I was so impressed by all that she knew and did at her age.

I can recall one Christmas we did not have any money, there were no gifts under the tree. Our mom said that there was a Christmas party at the local Elks Lodge, and we were all invited, the six of us scrambled in my mom's car, squealing with excitement at going to a Christmas party. As we pulled up to this large, impressive stone building, I thought how beautiful it looked with all the snow and lights, there was a large wreath on the door with a red bow. I could not wait to enjoy this evening with my siblings.

We entered the front door, the smell of baked ham waft through the air, one of my all-time favorites. I could not remember the last time we all got to have ham! We were ushered to our seats and given a nice hot meal, followed by chocolate cream pie, my god I thought I was in heaven. I had no idea how my mom snagged us invites but I was so happy I could barely contain myself. I was not the only one feeling this way, there were so many kids here running around, all so excited about the party and what surprises the night may bring.

After our meal we were ushered into a large auditorium, the youngest was to start filling in at the front and the oldest towards the back. An older lady took to the stage and introduced herself as Belle Davis, she had white hair and the cutest rhinestone glasses. I remember her walking around during dinner making sure each of us had enough to eat and drink. Belle was explaining that shortly each of us would be going to Santa's Workshop, and we would be allowed to pick out one toy for ourselves. I honestly did not think my day could have gotten any better but after hearing that I was like "Wow!"

    They started calling out the age groups, I patiently waited to hear my group which was number 5. The kids were so excited they were running up the stairs as they were called. I smiled as they came back down the stairs with their gift from Santa's Workshop, smiling from ear to ear with excitement. "Okay, all 5-year old's, please walk this way to Santa's Workshop." It was finally my turn; I was moving at a fast pace.

    I approached the top of the stairs, there was this enormous room filled with toys from wall to wall. I had never seen so many toys in my entire life. I knew exactly what I wanted, a doll, the tall kind with the long hair that you could brush. My eyes glanced up and down the isles looking for her, as I turned around to check the other side of the room, I spotted her, leaning against a baby-doll highchair, wearing a baby blue dress, blue bow in her hair with white shoes. She was exactly what I remember seeing in the toy book from Montgomery Wards. I found her! The butterflies in my stomach were going crazy as I ran over to where she was. I grabbed Ms. Lolly Dolly up and off we went to proudly display it to all those that were watching as I bound down the stairs. I do not know if I floated down those stairs, but I couldn't recall coming down them.

    I remember just being so happy, I wanted to find my brothers and sister and show them my brand-new baby-doll. I spotted them, a couple of rows back from my seat "hey, look, look it's that baby-doll from the catalog!" I could see my older brother Scott smiling but also gesturing for me to sit down at the same time. I know they were going to be just as happy as I was once, they entered that room upstairs and saw all the toys to choose from!

Yup, just as I thought, I watched each of my sibling's bop down the stairs with huge smiles plastered on their faces, feeling like they had just picked up the best gift ever! That day and every Christmas after, I will never forget the generosity shown to my family. The six of us left that Elks Lodge that day feeling like we were included, we were made a part of a very special event that changed all our adult lives forever.

As I got older, Evan and I would make monetary donations to local charities to help families in need during the holidays. Evan knew what it meant for a family to wake up and enjoy opening gifts, and I knew what it meant to wake up to no gifts at Christmas. As our children got a little older, I would take them out shopping for gifts to donate to local families. I remember the one year we were out shopping with the kids and Bryan picked out a small bike and helmet for the local charity, he was only about 8-years old at the time. When we arrived at the drop off location, Bryan hopped out of the truck with Evan, he pushed that bike into the garage beaming from ear to ear knowing that some young boy would be getting that bike for Christmas. Hailey always picked out cool trendy gifts, one year, it was an iPod. She wanted to give them something that she knew was popular at the time and all the other kids at school had it.

To this day, both of my kids are very caring, thoughtful adults. Evan instilled so much in both of our children, to always show kindness and caring to those less fortunate. Without Evan I think I would still be clinging to being the best based out of what my ego was telling me at the time.

Me, I want to be like Beth!

To look back at Beth now, that girl had her shit together! She did not care about impressing others, she would walk out of her house with her hair up in a ponytail. She would slip on her husbands oversized football jersey and slip into her old sneakers, she was all about comfort. You would not find one stich of brand name items on her or in her wardrobe! Believe me, Beth could afford it, but her priority in life was her family. Her time and energy were focused on them, not a false persona.

You would find Beth still hanging out with her loyal girlfriends from high school. They were all like sisters, their bond could never be broken. Their close friendship was of trust and supporting each other. Her home was lived in, and the family's scruffy dog lay sprawled out near the fireplace. The kids ran around laughing, all wired up on sugar. There was no judgement, there was no one upping each other, and no materialistic egos to deal with!

So many years after high school Savanah was still giving it her all to keep up with appearances. She still looked as beautiful as ever, not a hair out of place. She had a new circle of friends that looked just as magnificent as her. Her home was clean and spotless, like a museum. Her children went to the finest schools that she could afford. She certainly appeared to be living her best life ever!

I wanted to continue to stay grounded, I did not want to lose myself, while trying to please everyone else. I was going to live my life exactly the way I wanted to live it. The first thing I did was kick Ego's ass out the door, it was no longer going to occupy space in my brain. The second thing I did was start cleaning out my closet. All those things I started buying thinking, "This will make me happy!" that and so many other things were packed up in a box and donated to Good Will. It was painful parting with name brand items, not because I felt I could not live without them. I hated the fucking fact that I spent so much money on them! I had been suckered into a society that made me feel that material things had so much value in life.

For me that thought process was very difficult to separate. The poor girl still felt I needed material things, the widow felt buying new things always made her happy. Then we had the realistic widow that said, "None of this material shit means anything. I could replace it all if I had to. The living, breathing people in my life cannot be replaced!" I felt the realistic widow had the best advice! I know the therapist had a lot to do with the way the realistic widow was thinking.

Don't get me wrong, there are many talented artists out there that deserve the high dollars for their valued creations. But this black canvass bag I dragged out of my closet, what was I thinking, 4,000.00 dollars! Why? On that same shelf are three more black bags that look exactly alike. Some of the bags still had tags on them, the shoes only worn once! I was a freaking nightmare, shopping, buying, happy, happy. Ugggghhhhh not!

I started putting anything with a value over one hundred dollars in a separate box, labeled "Consignment" at least I was hoping I could get something back out of my frivolous happy spending. I had that box overflowing within two hours. There was stuff in there I had not worn or even looked at in years. It was all going out to consignment to be recycled back into the world at a lower price to someone that actually needed it.

The day I dropped my stuff off at the consignment store I walked around as they sorted through my things. I looked at the clothes hanging on the racks and was so taken aback by the quality of the items and the price. I was the girl that always shopped and paid full price for everything. To see these beautiful clothes set at a reasonable price captured my attention. I made a promise to myself from here on out, shopping would be at consignment shops. I was no longer going to be the person dropping off something to consignment that I had paid full price for.

As I walked out the door the nice lady at the consignment store said, "Mrs. Mills, we have a few items that we can't take." I replied, "Please give them to Good Will." I was cleaning out; I did not want to bring anything back home with me! I wanted the stuff gone; I wanted the clutter cleared out of my house! I know this sounds strange but shit, I think this whole decluttering thing was helping me with my anxiety. I could sit in my home without feeling claustrophobic from all the stuff. I could open my closet door and not feel the guilt of all my spending sprees.

I started feeling better working on me! It felt like I was shedding old skin. All that I was doing felt right to me. I no longer felt the need to put makeup on or do my hair if I was leaving my home. I would take a shower; comb my hair and I was off to start my day. I did not care about impressing people. I did not feel the need to want people to like me.

    I had a new circle of friends our friendships were effortless. I had new hobbies and was doing things that I enjoyed. My love for landscaping and working outside now occupied my time. I stayed away from negative energy and toxic people; I was breathing a whole new life into me. I had lost so many friends and family members, all of them preferred the old Mallory. The new Mallory wanted peace in her life, the new Mallory no longer tolerated petty bullshit drama. It drove me crazy hearing "friends" talk about friends, and "family" talking about family. Where in the hell was the loyalty and the trust. I thought, hell, I was that person at one time that they were all talking about, now they have found another vulnerable victim.

    I cut these people off from my life, they had no clue how precious life was or how to be a genuine friend or family member. I wish them all the best in their life, but I could never foresee ever having a close relationship with them again. The emotional ups and downs of liking me or loving me one minute to hating me the next were over. The unbearable loss of Evan showed me to live a beautiful life today with no promise of another tomorrow.

    It was not easy climbing this mountain with so many obstacles in the way. There were days I just said, "the hell with it. I'm not trying today; I do not have the strength." The moment I started removing obstacles from my life, the rocks did not seem so slippery. I had the strength! I finally climbed that steep mountain full of slippery rocks. I had stumbled and fallen so many times. Not this time. I made it to the top with all the bumps, bruises, and bleeding fingertips. The "Mallory" I knew and loved was back, and she wasn't going anywhere!

I want to thank my kids for always being my biggest supporters! I love you!

Made in United States
North Haven, CT
01 March 2023

33321015R00102